To There and Back Again…

My Wife's Journey through Leukemia and a Bone Marrow
Transplant on the Wings of Hope and Heroes

Thomas M. Wonica

ISBN:
ISBN-13: 978-1987419641

DEDICATION

This book is dedicated to my wife Christine. Your courage is remarkable, your will unbreakable, and your hope and faith unbending. You are my hero. Thank you for making it home.

To our daughter Kailey, thank you for making us laugh. You are the first miracle of our life. Without you it would have been a much tougher road; the world a darker place.

To the doctors and nurses at Memorial Sloan Kettering Cancer Center, we're forever in your debt. You're a group of special people that I thank God for every day. Thank you for your care, kindness, and for curing my wife.

To Robert Browning, thank you from the bottom of my heart for saving Christine's life. You're a remarkable man and now, a good friend. You have a heart of gold.

To my in-laws, parents, brothers and sisters, the entire Care for Christine Support Network, and our team, Angels for Christine,

SMILE BECAUSE WE DID IT!

CONTENTS

Prologue   1

1   Leukemia Enters Our Life   5

2   What's a Bone Marrow Transplant?   10

3   Our Journey Begins (Again)   14

4   Plan B(MT)   18

5   The Not So Helpless Husband   21

6   Purpose   25

7   Research   27

8   "I Wonder How She Is."   29

9   The Care for Christine Updates   32

    The First Update   32

    Day 0: The Transplant   47

    Day 25: Homecoming   65

    Day 100: Major Milestone!   79

    One Year Cancer Free   111

    Thanksgiving to Remember   113

10   The Hero, Robert Browning   116

11   Closure   122

ACKNOWLEDGMENTS

I would like to thank everyone who helped write this book. I may have documented Christine's journey through her diagnosis, treatments, and recovery, but so many of you helped write each chapter including the most perfect ending we could have ever asked for.

My wife Christine and our hero, Robert Browning are the main "characters" in this story of success. They are the hope and inspiration that we need more of in the world. I wrote the words, but they lived the story.

Dr. Jakubowski, Lauren, Kerry, Elizabeth, and rest of the amazing staff at Memorial Sloan Kettering Cancer Center made this book possible with their care and support.

The members of our support system, the **Care for Christine Support Network** and our LLS Light the Night walk team, ***Angels for Christine***, stood by us through the entire journey. Together, we continue the fight against cancer. With thousands of dollars raised to help fund research and patient services, we will continue to help write successful chapters for other families.

God bless you all!

Prologue

My wife Christine was initially diagnosed with leukemia in 2002 but the days that document her recovery in this book take place after her relapse in 2003. That was the most difficult part of Christine's battle. She took a journey that no one should have to take.

The memory is one I will never forget; one that will both haunt and inspire me for the rest of my life. My wife looked at me with tears in her eyes as we drove along the Staten Island expressway. Our day trip to New Jersey was nothing more than a feeble attempt to take her mind off of what lay ahead. We were trying to make things feel "normal." We were looking for a distraction. It didn't take long to realize that it just wasn't working. It was easy to see by the expression on Christine's face that her mind was racing, filled with thoughts of worry and uncertainty. I sat in the driver's seat praying that there was more I could do for her.

Days earlier our entire family was propelled into a surreal world of despair. (That may sound dramatic, but it actually doesn't begin to capture the weight of it all.) There had been a message waiting on our answering machine for us when we arrived home from vacation. It was from

Christine's doctor.   The message itself was not alarming; the professionals at Memorial Sloan Kettering Cancer Center (MSKCC) are wonderful with that sort of thing; but there's so much the imagination can do to influence a person who has already been effected by cancer. Whether it was a defense mechanism or post-traumatic stress from Christine's initial diagnosis I cannot say, but I braced for the worst and prayed for the best. It wasn't long before I reached the doctor and confirmed our worst fears, Christine had relapsed after almost a year in remission from leukemia; more specifically, acute myelogenous leukemia (AML). After months of chemotherapy treatments, physical and emotional suffering, and 9 months of recovery, the disease that had invaded Christine's body had returned. Her prayers of being cured had not been answered.

After breaking the news to her as gently as I could, Christine wondered if God would ever answer her prayers. I feared that despite all of the love and care she would receive, that Christine would feel alone battling this disease; and when you're getting ready to fight for your life that's not the way you want to go into it.

As we passed through the EZ-Pass lane on the New Jersey Turnpike Christine looked at me and asked a simple, heart breaking question;

"Can we just keep going?"

"Can we just keep going?" I asked, confused.

"Yeah, why can't we just keep driving? We can keep going down I-95 all the way to Florida. We can get far away from here and everything will be better. Maybe it will work itself out. We just need to get away and forget this ever happened."

I could feel my emotions begin to overtake me. I couldn't blame her for feeling that way, but I tried to be as stern and as confident as possible. It was the only thing I could do to stop myself from breaking down.

"You know we can't do that. We need to get you better and then we can go anywhere we want. Don't worry, everything is going to be alright. You have a lot of people who need you. This is going to work out." I silently made the sign of the cross in my mind. As we drove on together, two partners in life, I shared a quick reference to _Thelma and Louise_ which drew a brief smile behind her tears (there was no way we were driving off a cliff!). In the back of my mind I knew I had to be right.

Although my words were always meant to make my wife feel better, to comfort her in times of need, I knew there was little I could say to truly make Christine feel like all would be well in the end. It seemed there was little that could make her find anything positive in our situation. The one constant exception however, was our daughter Kailey. At just over a year and a half years old she was, and still is, our pride and joy. Through it all, Kailey also became Christine's motivation. She wanted nothing more in the world than to get her treatments over with and be back home with her daughter. Christine wanted to be able to tuck her in at night, watch her grow up, and just be a mom to her little girl.

Christine knew that if the leukemia returned her treatment options would be limited. She was now trying to prepare herself for a very difficult and life threatening procedure called a Bone Marrow Transplant (BMT).

Christine had already gone through multiple rounds of chemotherapy and had been in remission for nine months after first being diagnosed. Those nine months of recovery were the best days of our lives up until that point. We had a small nine month taste of what we had missed while Christine was in the hospital during her initial treatments. Christine was now faced with the realization that she was going to have to miss even more time with her family. It was discouraging, frustrating, and a very scary moment for us all, but Christine had the weight of the world on her shoulders. It felt like there was very little anyone could do to lighten the load.

Christine was about to embark on the toughest journey of her young 29-year-old-life. She had more questions than answers and the available facts and statistics surrounding a BMT were scary to say the least. The survival statistics, side-effects from the treatments, and the number of risks associated with the transplant were overwhelming. We knew however, that it was the next step in her road to recovery. A transplant was the next step on the ladder to a cure from this disease, and we didn't have a lot of time before Christine would be back in the hospital for the procedure.

For months following Christine's transplant the road was a hard fought battle. She worked hard for every milestone and endured pain and suffering beyond imagine. She redefined courage on a daily basis. She had her ups and downs but was surrounded by love every step of the way. Looking back on Christine's recovery it is clear what saved her life - her courage and determination, the love and support of her family and friends, a group of extremely talented doctors and nurses, our daughter Kailey, and the bone marrow of a willing donor who anonymously gave of himself so that Christine could live.

Since Christine's initial diagnosis in March of 2002 her fight has continued on and will for years to come. Even without leukemia in her body, the impact of this traumatic life event weighs heavily on our minds. Not all scars are visible, but we hope and pray every day that they continue to fade over time.

What Christine accomplished is a remarkable achievement by any standard. She went through one of the most rigorous procedures and recovery in the medical world. She has faced obstacles and overcome tremendous odds to get where she is today – cured from leukemia. Christine's road has been an amazing chapter in the lives of many. The number of people she's inspired and touched with her bravery and determination is evidenced in the countless letters and e-mails she has received over the years. Her story has given hope to many who are fighting their own battles, whether it be with leukemia, other forms of cancer, or other diseases. Christine takes pride in how far she has come and now smiles in knowing she has the opportunity to live a full life, cancer free.

As Christine's "primary care giver" I witnessed the woman I love suffer through more than anyone should. I felt my role was to be strong, especially in front of Christine. The reality was that no matter how strong I acted, seeing the love I met in High School and grew up to marry put through such a test of mind and body was traumatizing. I needed an outlet and found one in writing. What turned into a form of self-prescribed therapy, I logged our days and nights. I wrote about Christine's ups and downs, her progress and setbacks. Looking back on the thoughts that flowed from my mind to the computer screen makes me smile because I was able to capture a series of amazing moments that now define a large part of who we are as a family.

I wrote this book for two primary reasons; to honor my wife's undying will to succeed in her fight against leukemia, and to share her story as an inspiration to those fighting battles in their own lives, regardless of what the obstacles might be.

This is the story of a remarkable woman's fight to survive cancer. This is my wife's story.

Chapter 1

Leukemia Enters Our Life

Leukemia hit our family like a thief in the night. It was totally unexpected and without warning. It's a disease, like countless others, that does not discriminate by age, sex or any other denomination. The exact cause of leukemia is unknown. There are factors that raise a person's chances of getting the disease such as exposure to benzene, a chemical found in cigarettes and various other products, but the explanation of how a person gets leukemia was interesting. I'll paraphrase the doctors' explanation with this, "[The body has a 'hiccup' and makes a mistake with a white blood-cell. That blood cell can lay dormant for a long period of time, sometimes never showing itself. In people with leukemia, that mistake of a cell comes alive and starts reproducing. It serves no function, but will reproduce and reproduce until there's no room for the good blood cells the body needs for carrying oxygen, clotting blood, and fighting disease and infection.]" In a nutshell and at a very high level, that's leukemia. Although the disease is prevalent in older people, usually those over 55 years of age, my wife is proof that there are no true age limits. Many of the patients that we met in the hospital are proof of the same. Leukemia does not discriminate.

Before Christine was diagnosed in March of 2002 it was a very exciting time for our family.

There was a lot going on all around us and we were moving and grooving with what seemed like all kinds of important tasks and events. In the first two weeks of March we moved into our new home. We had spent a significant amount of time renovating our house and we were excited to finally move in. We had walked through it a thousand times discussing the memories we would create within its walls.

Our daughter Kailey was seven months old. Christine was a very proud new mom and decided to surpass her goal of breast feeding for just the first six months because it had been going so well. Christine said it made her feel closer to Kailey.

I was set to start a new job on March 18th. It was a great new opportunity and a decision I made to better my career for my family's future. So much was going on, and all very exciting; a new house, a new job, our 'little bean' Kailey was still brand new and we had so many expectations.

Horror struck during the middle of March. Christine had noticed a lump in her breast while feeding Kailey and brought it to her doctor's attention. The doctor wasn't too concerned and thought it was a lactating fibroid, something common in women who breastfeed. He sent her for an MRI and the test confirmed what they thought to be two non-cancerous masses.

I went with Christine to a surgeon for her next check-up and the doctor was almost positive the masses weren't cancerous, but he wanted to remove them just to make sure. He checked his schedule and assigned Christine a surgery date for two weeks in the future. It was easy to see Christine was not comfortable with the two week wait so we asked the doctor if he could do anything to move the date closer. I explained that the stress of the unknown was keeping her up at night and Christine expressed concern in having to wait that long. Honestly thinking there would be little that he could do, Dr. Lansigan picked up the phone right there in the examination room and scheduled Christine's surgery for the very next day. He made the change for Christine's peace of mind and we were extremely grateful, but we had no idea just how important that two week shift to an earlier date actually was. Whether it was divine intervention or just a really compassionate doctor, or both, that extra two weeks quite possibly saved Christine's life.

I took Christine to the hospital early the next day for 'pre-op'. It was March 15, 2002. I felt badly for her because of how extremely nervous she was about the procedure. She had been reassured by the doctor that it was a standard procedure and that it would hardly leave a scar. To ease both our minds we made plans to go out to dinner that night. I was planning on taking her somewhere special since we expected local anesthesia and thought Christine would be fine in time for dinner. I still recall the last words I said to her before she left me in the waiting room that morning, "Don't worry babe, I'll be waiting right here when you get out. You're going to be fine. I promise." Those final two words still ring in my ears.

There was no way I could have known what was to happen. As the saying goes, 'hindsight is 20/20' and the whole situation makes a little more sense now; why my vibrant, energetic, and athletic wife was so tired and out of breath as we moved out of our apartment and into our new home; why she had so many black and blues the day after we moved; why her breast milk had started to dry up unexpectedly although she was feeding Kailey regularly. These were all signs of what we were to find out, not from the surgery, but from the pre-surgery blood work.

When the operation was complete, Christine's doctor came in to get me from the waiting room. He was with another doctor I didn't recognize. As they rounded the corner and came into the room I could tell from their faces that something was wrong. I could feel the smile melt away from my face as I walked over to meet them. Dr. Lansigan looked as if he had seen a ghost. The other doctor looked only slightly more composed. Dr. Lansigan, with very little color left in his face, told me that the masses they removed from Christine's breast were not cancerous. I pre-maturely started to breathe a sigh of relief until I realized there was more.

"Mr. Wonica, we may have a different problem. Christine's blood work came back abnormal from the lab. Her CBC didn't look right."

A CBC or 'complete blood count,' measures a number of parts in the blood such as the count of the various blood cell types. In Christine's case, her red, white and platelet cell counts were not what they should be and the white counts were way off.

"What do we do now?"

"We are re-running the tests in the lab now because, honestly, your wife looks too good physically for the results to be hers. It may have been a mistake in the lab."

"What could it mean if the test results are not a mistake?" I asked.

"These types of readings usually indicate a blood disorder of some kind."

"What kind of blood disorder?"

"We usually see this with leukemia or lymphoma."

I crumbled to the hospital floor.

My world went dark.

From that point on our life changed. The "important" things we were dealing with at home; the house, the job, everything outside of my wife's illness, were no longer as important. The only thing that mattered at that moment was the health of my wife, Kailey's mom.

Breaking the news to Christine was the hardest thing I have ever done in my life. When the new blood tests came back showing the same abnormality, she was in post-op recovery and had no idea what was happening. As far as Christine knew we still had dinner reservations. She didn't know she needed help. I chose not to tell her right away. I called our parents and asked them to meet us at the hospital as quickly as they could. When they arrived Christine immediately became uneasy. She could tell something was wrong. It was at that moment that I explained to her that she was going to spend some time in the hospital while the doctors looked closely at her blood. I explained that the results of her blood tests had come back abnormal. She asked me the same question I had asked the doctor, "What could it mean?" I told Christine what I knew and with one conversation, one visit to the hospital for what was supposed to be a routine out-patient surgery, we began the most important journey of our life.

Within the next week, through a series of events, traumatizing experiences, and with the help of Dr. Mahmoud Aly, an amazing onsite hematologist, we found ourselves in one of the best cancer hospitals in the world; Memorial Sloan Kettering Cancer Center (MSKCC). In less than one week from that fateful day, Christine checked into the leukemia and lymphoma unit of one of the best cancer centers in the world.

Sloan was a big difference from the hospital we had left. From the moment we stepped out of the ambulance I could feel the difference. The nurses were exceptional and we were greeted by a staff that immediately raised our level of confidence. It was my wife's life we were fighting for and MSKCC had a whole floor dedicated to fighting blood cancer.

Christine's blood samples had made their way to the doctors at MSKCC prior to our arrival and it wasn't long before Christine was officially diagnosed with acute myelogenous leukemia (AML), a blood cancer affecting her white blood cells. Christine was immediately given a room on the 12th floor, where blood cancer patient resided, surrounded by an expert staff of doctors and nurses. Not more than a day after her arrival, Christine's first round of chemotherapy began. It was called her induction round, to be followed by four rounds of consolidation chemotherapy, a type of maintenance.

During her first treatments Christine, her parents, and I were in and out of the hospital on a regular basis while my parents took care of Kailey at our home so she would be comfortable while we were away. I started my new job a week later than expected, knowing full well we would need the medical benefits once the bills started rolling in. I fought hard to deal with reality in the midst of the surreal, while Christine fought for her life. The induction round of chemotherapy was an adventurous two months in the hospital that could fill a book on its own. The four additional rounds of chemo were a week of in-patient procedures followed by almost daily trips into the hospital for medication, check-ups and blood transfusions. We quickly learned that fighting a disease like leukemia was not a true science, and although the hospital and medical community had come a long way in understanding this disease, there were no guarantees. Everyone was different in the treatments they could tolerate and how they reacted to different medication. We did our best not to look too much at the statistics associated with the various treatments, and Christine relied on me to filter out the 'need to know' information and give it to her a little softer than a medical professional might. They had a responsibility to disclose everything, but given Christine's increased anxiety she didn't necessarily need to know everything, especially if the medication wasn't optional.

We were blessed and extremely fortunate that Christine went into remission after her induction round of chemo. She stayed in remission through the consolidation rounds as well, but there were some difficult decisions made along the way.

One of the first difficult decisions we had to make was whether or not to go forward with a Bone Marrow Transplant (BMT) or to rely on chemotherapy treatments alone for a cure. We researched the transplant, something we had heard of but knew very little about. Christine relied on me to collect all the necessary information so she could make a decision. I looked inside myself, to the doctors, nurses, medical journals, books, and the internet for answers and recommendations. We even sought medical advice from another prestigious cancer hospital. Christine and I discussed her options and she asked me to help her make a decision. I firmly believe the path we chose together, as husband and wife standing side by side, contributed a great deal to saving her life.

Chapter 2

What's a Bone Marrow Transplant?

There's no guarantee that someone will be in remission after a chemotherapy treatment. Remission meant the cancer was no longer presenting in Christine's blood. If the cancer comes back after remission, called a relapse, there's even less of a chance of someone going into remission a second time. Leukemic cells can potentially build up a tolerance to chemotherapy and may not react the same way a second or third time. As a matter of fact, with every relapse, remission would become more difficult to attain. So, it was a happy day indeed when Christine's blood test results after her induction round of chemotherapy came back telling us that she was in remission. The doctor could see no leukemia cells under the microscope and the more extensive cytogenetic tests, which look at the white blood cells' chromosomes, came back negative as well.

This was a great start for us and we knew that although there was a chance there were undetected leukemia cells in her body, there was a good chance that the additional chemotherapy rounds would be a great way to attack relentlessly and destroy them.

Shortly after Christine went into remission, we were shocked to hear Christine's doctor mention the potential need for a BMT. "A BMT!?!? But my wife is in remission!" The questions started flooding my mind.

"Her leukemia is gone, isn't it?" "What is a BMT anyway?" "How difficult of a procedure is it?" "Why does she need a transplant"?

I immediately got the itch to do some more research. I had already heard from nurses and other doctors that the transplant was a very difficult procedure and that it was extremely hard on the body. I collected the books I could get from the hospital and began reading. My mission was to learn as much as I could about the transplant and give Christine the 'book report' version of the procedure so she could decide what to do next. I searched the internet every chance I had to review the never-ending supply of information, just as I had done when she was first diagnosed.

I had often wondered how the doctors performed a procedure that replaced a person's bone marrow. Do they slice open the bones and scrape it out? Do they suck it all out with a big needle and then pump the new marrow in? I could not imagine how the procedure took place. Honestly, at that time I'm not sure I even really knew what bone marrow was let alone how to "transplant" it. What I found, after some reading, was that a BMT was a lot different than an organ transplant; take an organ out and then put a new one in. There was no bone cutting or bone replacement, but the details I read scared me.

I remembered back to when I spoke with a woman during Christine's hospital stay who was going through chemotherapy in preparation for a BMT. She asked me if Christine was going to have the procedure and I told her we didn't know yet. The woman went on to explain what she was going to go through. Of the whole story, I remember one part vividly. She said, "Before the transplant they bring you close to death with radiation and chemotherapy. It kills off your immune system and your body's ability to make its own blood. Then they give you the new bone marrow and the new immune system follows."

"Close to death." It would be an understatement to say that those words scared me.

I needed to read more about the side effects. I read about the things Christine *might* suffer and the things she would *definitely* endure. There were so many negative side effects covered in the books that my head started spinning; nausea, hair loss, sterility, forgetfulness, sluggishness, hormone loss, skin changes, eye problems, and the list continued on. It was also highlighted that some patients can't physically handle the procedure and pass away, not from leukemia but from the transplant. I had gotten used to the hospital staff telling their patients everything about procedures, including the risks. I had been Christine's buffer. I had to deliver this news to her in some shape or form and I didn't take the responsibility lightly. She was counting on me to tell her what she needed to know, and I needed to be sure of the information. Christine would make her decision based on the information I provided. Her doctor recommended a BMT while others did not. The final decision would not be easy.

Along the way we sought a second opinion from MD Anderson hospital in Seattle. A very nice doctor at MD Anderson agreed to review Christine's case. After reviewing he agreed that Christine had a fair chance that chemotherapy alone could cure her disease and a decision not to immediately undergo the transplant was viable. Armed with that information and the knowledge of what a transplant would bring, Christine made the final decision to not attempt the transplant. We'd keep it as 'Plan B'. We would hope that five rounds of chemotherapy, 1 induction round and four consolidation rounds (our 'Plan A') would be enough to cure her. We made the decision to hold off and keep the option on the shelf should, God forbid, Christine relapse. The transplant division at MSKCC had already started the search for a donor, a difficult process in itself, so they put their search on hold. We would wait and pray that Christine's remission held and that the leukemia would never returned. Christine's doctor supported our decision, and our 'Plan A' treatment and recovery carried on.

The months that followed Christine's final round of chemotherapy were amazing. We began to get our lives back on track. As individuals and as a family we started anew. We realized how much life had to offer and we vowed to grasp every moment and make the most of every second. Holidays were more meaningful, vacations more special, our time together felt even more precious.

There was always a little voice in the back of Christine's mind asking the tough questions, "Will the leukemia come back? Is it really gone forever?" Before and after each and every bone marrow biopsy, the test which searched her blood for signs of leukemia, massive waves of anxiety would come over her. She would feel the weight of the world back on her shoulders and it would remain there until her doctor told her she was still in remission.

By the ninth month, about four month after Christine's final round of chemotherapy, she felt great about her progress. We took a vacation with friends to the New Jersey shore and spent a wonderful time with our daughter by the beach. The world seemed a little brighter for us that summer and we continued to count our blessings for Christine's progress and continued good health.

Chapter 3

Our Journey Begins (Again)

We returned home from vacation without a care in the world. We had spent the week in Wildwood Crest, NJ enjoying the sun, the beach, the swimming pool and the amusement park. Christine and I thoroughly enjoyed watching our now two-year-old daughter Kailey go round and round on the carousel, mini-cars and baby-boats. Her smile had been worth the cost of the trip ten-fold and Christine and I never knew how wonderful it could be, how satisfying, to watch someone else have so much fun.

With the memory of Christine's recent battle against leukemia pushed as far back in our minds as it would let us, we were beginning to get back to 'normal,' except normal was now so much better than it ever was before. Each and every day was a gift and, more importantly, we realized it.

During the nine months of remission, Christine's hair had grown back, her immune system was back in full swing and there were times her whole bout with blood cancer seemed like it was just a bad dream. We held hands and hugged more often. Kailey was finally used to waking up with mommy and daddy home where we belonged. Everything was falling into place. We were getting our lives back.

As we pulled down the final stretch of roadway on our way home, we passed my parents' house on Perry Avenue. Not having seen my mom and dad for a while we decided a surprise visit was in order. We pulled up with our loaded car, got out and began our visit. We were there for roughly 15 minutes when I decided to bring the car to our house just up the road, unload the luggage and then return to finish the visit. I pulled into our dirt driveway and began the mundane task of taking everything into the house.

I opened the door for the first time in a week, and despite the stale hot air which escaped past me in the doorway, it was good to be home. It took six trips to the car to unpack everything. I remember thinking, "we should really cut back next time and travel lighter," something I reminded myself after every trip with Christine and Kailey. Finally, after everything was inside, I went into the kitchen to grab a drink from the fridge. I poured a glass of cold water and noticed the blinking light on the message machine.

I left the glass on the table and walked over to press 'play.' There were a few messages on the machine but only the first one is etched in my memory. The message was from Christine's doctor. It was short and to the point, "Mr. Wonica, this is Dr. Jakubowski, please give me a call back. It's important."

I registered her words for a moment. "Mr. Wonica," she said. As I mentioned earlier, I usually took all news and filtered it to Christine so a call to me was totally normal.

But what could be so "important"?

The message could have been about anything, but I could feel a lump begin to swell in my throat along with a growing knot in my belly. I saw spots before my eyes and the world began to spin. Confusion and uncertainty joined me in the kitchen and panic began to set in.

"Please no...Please no," I repeated to myself as I picked up the phone and dialed the number to the hospital, which I now knew by heart. Because it was Sunday, I reached the hospital's answering service and told the operator I needed to speak with the doctor. I explained the message and my wife's situation. After a few minutes I was put in touch with the on-call physician. I was told I'd have to call back on Monday to speak with Christine's doctor who was not on-call. I was adamant, almost pleading that her doctor be paged. The message said, "It was important." I couldn't wait until Monday to find out about my wife's health; her life. It took a little coaxing but I eventually found myself pacing the kitchen, praying and waiting for the doctor's call. Time seemed to stand still for those 10 or so minutes. Then the phone rang. I picked it up.

"Hello?"

"Hello Mr. Wonica," said the doctor.

"Hi doctor." I wanted to scream, "Please don't tell me it's back!"

"We saw something under the microscope from Christine's last blood test that doesn't look normal. We have to wait for the results of the chromosome tests to be 100% positive, but it looks like Christine's leukemia is presenting once again."

My body and mind went numb as I stood there dumbfounded. I pictured my wife down the block with Kailey, smiling, not knowing that we were going to have to start this all over again. The thought still breaks my heart.

Without thinking, I asked myself out loud, "How do I tell her? I already had to do this once. How do I tell her again? What do we do now?"

The doctor, God bless her, was to the point immediately, "You're going to calm down and be strong. You're going to get Christine in here first thing tomorrow morning and we're going to start making her better. We begin preparing for a BMT and beat this thing once and for all."

I hung up with Christine's doctor, shaking with fear and frustration. I just couldn't take my mind from Christine's smiling face and the understanding that for the second time in less than a year I would have to tell my beautiful, loving wife that she was going to have to enter a fight for her life.

I stood in our dining room thinking out my next steps. I was paralyzed with sympathy and fear. Sympathy for the woman I loved and fearful she would simply give up after already having traveled such a long road with this disease. How do you go from a wonderful family vacation to fighting leukemia all over again in a matter of seconds? Five more minutes passed and I heard a light knock on the door.

My dad walked in, looking to see if I needed any help unpacking. He took one look at my face. "What's wrong?"

"I just got off the phone with the doctor…" was all I could get out before I broke down. He hugged me and that comfort allowed me to compose myself. It was only my father and I in the room at that moment. I needed that hug to be able to move on and support my wife. I knew how much it broke his heart to see his son going through this with his family; a disease like this affects the whole family. Parents are often so used to being able to pull their family through any situation;

but when even a father or mother does not have the answers, sometimes a hug goes a very long way to helping get someone back on track. It may have been my saving grace that day.

It wasn't long after my father entered that I heard footsteps on the porch. I had already regained my composure and wiped my eyes dry before her smile walked into the dining room. I'll never make it as an actor because with one look my wife's smile was replaced with something else.

The next few hours can easily be called one of the most difficult and trying moments of our entire life together as a couple. As horrible as it was, it can also be viewed as one of the things that has brought us even closer in our relationship, something I would have said was impossible. At that moment it felt like we needed each other more than ever. It was the definition of "for better or for worse; in sickness and in health." We look forward to the "better" and the "health," even take it for granted, but it's the "worse" and "sickness" of that sacred vow that can make us stronger in our relationships; stronger in love. It is through that adversity that we can become stronger in life together. Wedding vows, and their true meaning are absolutely amazing. They are not just words. They are powerful and important, and we must be prepared to honor them when the time comes. Unfortunately, that time will most likely arrive unannounced. It comes when we least expect it. It may even ruin your post-surgery dinner plans or a family vacation.

In the time after I told Christine the bad news there was a lot of crying and a lot of hugging. As our families came together, rallying around us with support, there was a tremendous amount of love displayed, which immediately filled the hole left by despair. There are few words that can explain the immediate impact of the situation. It can be figuratively likened to an unexpected punch in the gut by a heavyweight fighter, but so much worse. It was shortly after that phone call with the doctor that I knew we were going to need a lot of help from our family and friends. We would need all the prayers we could get. We would undoubtedly need blood donations and a lot of positive energy. I immediately started thinking about a new plan of attack.

Before Christine even began to prepare to leave our daughter for more time in the hospital; before Christine started thinking about what a BMT would mean for her and her family, she looked up at me with big, blue, tear filled eyes and asked, "Tommy, what are we going to do now?"

I took her in my arms and stared deep into her eyes, and spoke with a sincere confidence, "We're going back into the hospital to make you better." The doctor's words just had to be right.

Chapter 4

Plan B(MT)

The next few days were spent traveling back and forth to MSKCC to get ready for Christine's next round of chemo, a preparatory round before the transplant would take place. The game plan was simple, although actually getting to the end-point would not be. Christine would go through a single round of chemotherapy to try and get her back into remission. Given the past results of former transplant patients, we knew that remission would put Christine in a better position for a successful transplant. After a single round of chemotherapy, Christine would go in for a BMT if MSKCC's bone marrow donor search could find a donor whose blood "matched" Christine's. The donor would also need to agree to make the sacrifice of donating their stem cells or bone marrow. We held our breath anxiously awaiting the results of Christine's chemotherapy round. We really wanted her back in remission, but as I mentioned before, we knew it would be more difficult to achieve this time around. So, our family prayed while the doctors, nurses, and staff at Sloan went to work.

Through the whole process to this point, Christine and I quickly became what I call 'non-medical' experts on BMTs. I had read and reviewed all the facts that I could find and reviewed the information with Christine. We were thankful 'Plan A' bought Christine nine months of recuperation during her first remission, but we now dove head first into Plan B(MT) knowing full well it would be much more difficult this time around. Our goal with 'Plan A' was to find a cure while avoiding a transplant. We knew from our original rounds of chemo that Christine, most likely, had an unrelated donor out there someplace who would be considered a "perfect match". A "perfect match" means that someone in this great wide world had blood with a set of critical chromosomes that matched Christine enough for a transplant to not only be possible, but favorable. In fact, initial searches had turned up someone whose bone marrow matched Christine's. We needed to reconfirm this and the donor would have to be located and AGREE to participate in potentially saving Christine's life. You might think it would be a 'no brainer' for someone to make this decision, but it's a big commitment for the donor. The donor needs to take time out of their life to take medication, donate marrow or stem cells and recover from the procedure. This would take time away from family and work and also takes a physical toll on the donor's body, all for a total stranger. As the hospitals and donor centers started to work out the logistics it seemed like an awful lot of puzzle pieces to put together. Then our overactive brains began to take over. We started to worry. What if the contact information of the donor was incorrect and they couldn't find him or her? What if the donor simply said, "No?" What if they really weren't a match and the blood work was a mistake? We tried our best to keep our worries at bay and we hoped and prayed it would all come together. We put all our faith in the professionals who work with the blood donor centers around the world that the National Marrow Donor Program[1] would help save Christine's life.

Thank God that after two of the longest months of our life, MSKCC, the National Marrow Donor Program and the blood collection site of the matching donor worked out the logistics and the donor was lined up. From what we learned, which was very little, the donor was very excited to help us and that he was in fact a "perfect" match for Christine. There are rules around not being able to learn a donor's identity so we didn't know much else about him. We took that in stride and didn't worry. An anonymous donor it would be; at least for now.

Now that the donor details were straightened out and the transplant was as close to definite

---

[1]Official website can be found at http://www.bethematch.org

as it would be short of receiving the blood, we started to worry about the next, most crucial part of the procedure. It wasn't necessarily the radiation or chemotherapy that worried us. The most difficult part of the process would begin after those treatments as Christine deteriorated from their effects and then worked to recover.

Christine's recovery would be critical and entail a list of rules and guidelines a mile long for both Christine and those around her to strictly follow. Recovery would require Christine and I, as well as our entire contingent of family and friends to be as diligent as possible in keeping her out of harm's way. We would all play a crucial role in her recovery. For a few, it would mean physically being there and helping. For many others, the help would be in forcing themselves to physically stay away, but offer support through writing letters and e-mails. For Christine, it would mean fighting each and every day for her life.

It didn't seem fair. My wife was looking and feeling as good as ever, but simultaneously preparing to intentionally get very sick as the chemotherapy and radiation treatment dates approached. So, as Christine and I sat and ran through the series of steps to get her to a cure, we realized very quickly, it was going to get a whole lot worse before it got better.

Chapter 5

The Not So Helpless Husband

As Christine prepared for the fight of her life, I prepared for another stint of being the most supportive husband I could be. I vowed to stay by her side as often as needed until she was well again. I feared, however, that other than being there for her there was little else I could do. I began to feel helpless and tried hard to stay as upbeat as possible in order to fight off depression. I thought long and hard about how to make a greater impact on her recovery.

You can imagine the feeling of helplessness that ran through me at not being able to save my wife; to solve this problem for her. I had gotten used to being the husband who could pull our family through anything. I enjoyed being the man of the family and taking on those responsibilities. I enjoyed starting to be that type of father. It made me proud to be able to take care of my family and provide them a good life. It might sound absurd, but it broke my heart that I was not able to deliver my wife from this illness and make her well again.

Beginning with Christine's visit to the hospital in March of 2002 I had a number of conversations with God. Before Christine's relapse I tried to negotiate deal after deal, promising everything I could think of to just make and keep her better. Those conversations started again after her relapse. I prayed for guidance and for inspiration in addition to praying for Christine's health. I knew deep down that if I let our situation bring me down I would bring Christine down as well. I couldn't let that happen.

As I reflected on the procedure Christine was preparing for, there was a short period of a few hours that I'll just call my "rough period." Although it was not easy, I took a good, honest look inside myself for answers. I could play the hopeless victim, or I could try and make a difference in any way I could. After those few hours alone I pulled myself together and once again focused on that vow Christine and I took on July 24, 1999: "in sickness and in health." It was then I realized that I'd already made my deal with God on our wedding day. I knew the only thing I could do was be there for her, by her side, and continue to take on this disease with her. We had agreed that although Christine would be bearing the physical brunt of the disease, it wasn't just her with leukemia. 'We' had leukemia and we'd fight it together.

It was shortly before Christine went into the hospital for the BMT that a light bulb went off in my head. I finally thought of a way to help Christine fight day in and day out; a way to cope with the days, weeks, and possibly months away from our daughter and the rest of the outside world. Christine needed to know that she wasn't alone; consistently reminded that she was not alone. When the going got tough, she needed to be reminded that we loved her; that a lot of people loved her and that we were pulling for her every step of the way.

I thought back to the first five rounds of chemotherapy Christine went through. I especially remembered the initial induction round where she spent almost two months in the hospital without coming home. I saw similarities to what she would experience during her transplant, but a few things stood out:

1) During induction Christine was able to visit Kailey in the lobby of the hospital because children weren't allowed on the leukemia floor, but Christine was allowed out of her room. This time, Chrissy would be without any interaction with Kailey for the entire duration of her hospital stay. She wouldn't be allowed to leave her hospital room for 5-8 weeks and Kailey wouldn't be allowed up to the room.

2) During her induction and consolidation rounds of chemotherapy, Christine was able to have as many visitors as she wanted as long as we were strict about those

who posed a health risk with colds and illnesses. This was excellent considering so many people came by to offer support and pay a visit. This time Christine would not be able to see anyone but her doctors, nurses, parents and me.

3) During her induction and consolidation rounds of chemotherapy it was easy for people to stay updated on Christine's progress by stopping by for a visit or by calling her room. We were easily able to communicate her status and ask people for help when we needed it. This time, the procedure would be much more intense. Christine would find it difficult to get out of bed some days and recovery would be much slower than before. She would need the help of her mom, dad and me as much as possible. Our focus would be on Christine. There would be very little time for us to contact the many people wondering how she was doing.

4) As with the first rounds of chemotherapy, blood donations would be a must. As a matter of fact, the need for whole blood and platelet donations would be even greater during the more intense BMT. I needed a way to communicate this to our friends and family; strangers if need be. Christine's life might depend on it.

Those four items alone were reasons to take the next steps to help us get through her treatment. Christine's parents, my parents, and our friends and family began collecting contact information for what would be the foundation of the Care for Christine Support Network. I then created an e-mail address for our fight, CareForChristine@yahoo.com [no longer active]. Then came the website, http://CareForChristine.com to regularly update our support network with Christine's status. It would be the equivalent of our 'blog' before blogs were a thing. We would use that same list of contacts to solicit blood donations and prayers for Christine. We would remind people frequently that my wife, their friend, cousin, sister, niece, acquaintance, former team-mate, and colleague was fighting for her life and needed all the support they could muster. The idea was simple, but I was proud of it. To our delight and surprise, the Care for Christine Support Network was a success and it became an important part of Christine's recovery.

It didn't take us long to find out there were a lot of people out there who wanted to be a part of our fight. Our initial list of supporters quickly grew from a few dozen into the hundreds. People started to forward our e-mails to friends and they forwarded them on to friends of their own.

Many wanted to help; they wanted to make a difference; they wanted to do whatever they could for Christine. It was encouraging to say the very least. The outpour of support in the form of emails, website hits, blood donations and hand written letters of support was extremely emotional. The thought of how much support we received from family members right down to complete strangers still brings tears to my eyes. We were truly blessed.

During her fight, the CareForChristine.com website was updated regularly, e-mail updates were sent to our supporters, messages from friends and family were posted to our site as signs of encouragement for everyone involved, and visitors signed the Guest Book and sent e-mails regularly to wish Christine well and bring a smile to her face.

The impact of the messages Christine received cannot be measured with anything material, but can be summed up in one statement Christine made while in the hospital recovering from her transplant. After having read roughly 20 e-mail messages from our Care for Christine Support Mailbox with her head still on her pillow because she was too tired and weak to lift it, she raised her eyes to me and whispered through dry cracked lips, "I guess we're not fighting this thing alone." She even managed a small smile through the pain right before falling asleep.

Since the inception of the Care for Christine Support Network, dozens of updates were written, beginning with her pre-transplant chemotherapy and continuing right through each major milestone. The updates are both a reminder of my wife's hard fought battle against a tough disease and her fight to recover from an intense treatment. They are a journal of her days in and out of the hospital, as well as a celebration of her accomplishments. They are a peek into the mind of a husband who watched his wife fight for her life as he stood by her side giving the only things he could; love and support. The updates are a glimpse into the struggles of a family doing their best to keep up a fight forced on them by an unwelcome guest; leukemia.

Chapter 6

Purpose

Throughout the months and years following Christine's BMT, many people have reached out to us regarding her story and fight through recovery. She has helped to inspire and motivate people who are either battling illnesses of their own or watching loved ones travel similar journeys. Christine's story has helped others in their own time of need and has given people strength when they needed it most. Some of the most rewarding messages we have received are from people we have never met, facing some form of cancer or illness affecting their family. At some point they were either forwarded one of Christine's updates or the link to our website. In our story, they have found courage in our strength as a family and my wife as a patient, fighter, and survivor. Some have used it as inspiration to carry on.

It's a wonderful feeling for Christine, knowing she has been able to positively impact others through her bout with leukemia. Our greatest HOPE is that her story continues to help others in their own personal situations; that her story continues to inspire and motivate others to never give up in their own personal battles.

As you continue to read you will find that leukemia is more than just a disease that affects a person's white blood cells. It goes so much deeper than that. It attacks the mind, body, and soul. Although there are many factors that come into play with a BMT, our story gives you one perspective through the eyes of a family doing everything they can to win a war of life and death. We're excited and hopeful that it may be used by patients, their families, friends, and caregivers; that they may find inspiration to carry out their own fight against any barrier that stands in their way.

My wife isn't a famous person. She's not a celebrity selling her story because everyone wants a piece of her life. Christine is a mom, wife, daughter, sister, aunt, cousin, niece, and friend. She's the person who woke up one day to suddenly have her world turned upside down by an illness, never to be the same again. My wife is a good person. Christine is the everyday you and me. That's what makes her story so remarkable.

Chapter 7

Research

When someone you love prepares to fight a disease with such intense treatments its natural for loved ones to bury their faces in books and spend hours on the internet learning everything there is about what the patient is going to experience. "Who else has gone through it and what do they have to say about it?" Information can be very powerful. The first thing we all wanted to know, or were scared to find out, were the facts and statistics on the cure rates of BMTs. I found myself looking for the percentages for the success and failure of everything Christine underwent.

At some points it felt good to know the numbers and other times it made me want to cry. One thing that wasn't always clear as I read most of the articles and studies was the detail behind the tests. For example: Who was studied? How old were they? How many people were there? Who was running the study and what was the motivation behind it? Something I've learned through life is there are usually motivating factors behind any study made public. When one is performed and written about to the general public, they may be doing so to prove a specific point or influence an audience. The medical field is not impervious to this type of influence. So although statistics give us an idea at times, they may not always be disclosing all the necessary details. It's possible we're not getting the whole picture. It was with this realization that we took the information provided by studies in stride. We tried not to lose sleep over anything that wasn't positive. Eventually, we stopped looking at the studies all together. We had made out decision, and we were "all in."

Christine and I learned a great deal during our journey that began on March 15, 2002. For instance, after you've made the decision to go through a BMT, because it's the only hope for survival, all the studies and historical statistics in the world don't mean a thing. Only one statistic matters, and that's 100% success for the person you love. Win the battles. Win the war. Survive.

Chapter 8

"I Wonder How She Is"

The Care for Christine Updates, sent out via e-mail and posted on our website, were first meant to keep everyone on "the outside" aware of Christine's progress as she fought within the walls of MSKCC. It was the easiest way to distribute any kind of message in a flash. We hoped each and every message would carry news of progress and strides toward recovery. We also knew that if we needed to put out an emergency call for blood donations or other assistance, we could use it to spread the word. Over the course of time though, the updates took on a new meaning. We hadn't counted on the thousands of responses that filled the inbox.

With each and every update sent, dozens of responses found their way back, letting us know people were praying for us, that they were there for us in case we needed them. I can confidently say that without the updates, the level of positive energy flowing from the outside world into Christine's hospital room would not have been as high or impactful.

I had the honor of writing the updates on a regular basis. Day in and day out I tried my best to capture each significant moment of Christine's progress. I honestly felt that each update would help bring Christine closer to the next milestone. Inevitably, the updates also became my therapy, my outlet to relieve whatever stress and frustration I could shake loose from watching my wife suffer through her recovery. They allowed me to put down on paper what was going on around me and I let it flow freely from my mind and onto the computer screen. I let go of the anger, rage, helplessness, and frustration I felt in watching the woman I love fight for her life. Writing also let me focus on the important aspects of Christine's procedure by putting it all down on paper. It helped me know our exact situation and where we stood at any given time and, in turn, I helped Christine build her confidence as she prepared for each step of her battle. I usually answered the same questions in the updates:

- What was Christine's current status?

- What was next on the medical agenda and what had just passed?   And…

- What did all of this information actually mean?

More than a few times I included a personal note, or wrote to empty my mind and emotions. For me it beat crying in the hallways of the hospital, something that was still occasionally unavoidable despite the writing.

Ninety nine percent of the time I felt comfortable writing the updates, even excited at times. If I uncovered any doubts or something wasn't clear as my fingers typed away I sought guidance from a doctor or nurse to help fill the gaps.

The updates started not too long after Christine went into the hospital after her relapse. It was a time when the doctors and nurses worked to finalize the logistics around her transplant.

In the pages to follow, as you read through the updates, my hope is that you develop an understanding or even feel the same emotional pulls and pushes I felt sitting in the hospital writing them. The updates bring realism to what otherwise feels like a surreal chapter of our life.

So begins the story of Christine's journey through what could be considered one of the most difficult yet miraculous procedures in the world. The updates are a journal of my wife's journey since relapse; her fight through a BMT and her recovery thereafter. It is also a glimpse into the impact cancer has on the family as a whole, and the amazing things we can accomplish if we stick together. I've left each entry as original as possible by removing only minor pieces that didn't fit with the overall purpose of the passage. Where appropriate, I've included background information before the update to provide context and clarity to the information. I hope you find inspiration in their meaning as you join us on our journey.

Chapter 9

The Care for Christine Updates

I wrote our first update on September 27, 2003 shortly after Christine started her preparation for the transplant. The prep included chemotherapy, something she'd been through a number of times after first being diagnosed in March of 2002.

<u>Saturday, September 27, 2003:</u>

Christine was released from the hospital on Monday, September 23rd and has been home resting after her sole round of chemotherapy. Her blood counts are dropping and she is currently neutropenic, which means her immune system is significantly suppressed. She has gone for regular blood tests to monitor her red blood and platelet numbers.

We have learned that Christine's BMT is scheduled to begin roughly October 27th, with the actual transplant taking place in early November. Christine will be home unless she gets a fever. A fever would put her back in the hospital until her immune system comes back.

****

Chemotherapy was meant to knock Christine's white blood cells down to zero, but she would always need high enough red blood cells and platelets to survive. Regular doctor visits and blood tests were required after chemotherapy to ensure Christine's blood levels were safe.

Monday, September 29, 2003:

Christine visited the hospital this morning and her blood work showed her red blood and platelet counts were high enough to be released without transfusions.

She was rather uncomfortable today, suffering from a sore throat and a constant pain in the middle of her back, most likely caused by a medication she is taking. Her next doctor appointment is in the city on Wednesday morning. She is still neutropenic and cannot receive visitors other than immediate family. Christine's blood cell counts should start to rise in approximately 10 days. Her biggest problem so far is finding food that doesn't make her nauseous.

****

Nausea was one of the most common side effects for almost every part of Christine's treatments. Pain medication, anti-anxiety medication, anti-viral medication, anti-fungal medication, and even anti-nausea medication made her vomit.

Wednesday, October 1, 2003:

Christine is toughing out what should be the middle of her chemotherapy treatment. Her counts are still rather low and I would expect her next blood transfusions to take place either Thursday or Friday. It all depends how she feels. The visit should just be for blood transfusions and then we come back home.

Signs that Christine needs red blood cells include exhaustion and shortness of breath. The most tell-tale sign that she needs platelets are small purple blemishes called petechiae usually on her legs or in her mouth. They look like little un-raised blood blisters.

Christine's potential bone marrow donor is an unrelated male, whose "major" chromosomes matched Christine's 10/10. [10/10 or ten for ten, is the term describing a donor whose blood chromosomes favorably match a patient's making a BMT possible.

Anything less than 10/10 significantly increases the risk of complications for an already VERY risky procedure.] Finding a donor with such a match is an EXCELLENT first step in this process. We aren't allowed to know any more about the donor for at least 1 year according to the process. Christine will go into the hospital on October 27th to begin treatment for the BMT, with the actual transplant taking place in early November. (We hope he agrees to go through the donation!)

****

You learn a lot about someone through an illness like leukemia and its treatments. I knew when Christine needed blood transfusions; I knew when she was sad, happy, tired and depressed. I also learned just how brave she was all over again.

Thursday, October 2, 2003:

Yesterday, Christine had a great morning but began to feel tired and worn down toward mid-afternoon. Her breathing became labored and a headache came on later in the day. They had a saying in the hospital however, "uncomfortable at home sure as hell beats comfortable in the hospital." I think Christine agrees, but we still have to be cautious as her immune system will be compromised for at least another week.

Christine will undoubtedly need some type of blood transfusion on Friday, Oct. 3. Her appointment is for 8:30AM and should last well into the afternoon. Although it will be a long day, possibly requiring both red blood and platelets be given, it will hopefully give Christine the opportunity to spend the whole weekend relaxing with Kailey and I without having to make a trip into Urgent Care. Last Sunday we spent over 10 hours in Urgent Care and it was a little frustrating for her.

Christine has been a real trooper during this round of chemotherapy, and despite a very difficult time sleeping, she's hanging tough. Just to tell you how strong my little lady is; Christine is required to give herself a shot every night. Yes, a needle type shot. What makes it more impressive is that the shot is administered to the stomach region. She gives herself the shot as I try hard not to faint.

****

Allergic reactions or any reaction to medication or treatment were always something we were on the lookout for. Having received dozens of transfusions in the previous year and a half, Christine knew her body well enough to know right away if something didn't feel right. Usually, after we corrected the problems with the help of the nurses or doctors the only thing that still remained was a whole lot of anxiety.

<u>Friday, October 3, 2003:</u>

Christine had 2 more blood transfusions today, one for red blood and one for platelets. She experienced an allergic reaction to the platelet transfusion and required Benadryl to stop the reaction. She has had reactions to platelets in the past, most likely due to a "fast drip" on the IV. The Benadryl helped Christine get back to normal and the transfusion continued.

This allergic reaction consisted of shallow breathing, tightness in her chest, and hives. Other than anxiety, she was fine afterwards and noticed easier breathing after the red blood was given to her. We head into the weekend in good spirits.

****

You never get used to some of the side effects chemotherapy brings. As a man I can get used to a receding hairline and have the easy option to shave my head if I'm getting a little too bald up top. It's just not the same for a 29-year-old woman who loses her hair because of medical treatments. It's very tough to deal with both physically and emotionally. According to Christine, it was a constant reminder of the disease she had. It was also a reminder that she was in the fight for her life.

<u>Saturday and Sunday, October 4th and 5th, 2003:</u>

Christine's hair began to fall out on Saturday. She made the decision to cut her hair nice and short. Christine figured, "If it's going to happen, I'm going to do it, not the chemo."

As you can imagine, despite the good attitude, this part of the fight is never easy and there were some tears shed. They were short lived though, as Christine got the buzzer out and went to town on my head [a show of support]. Then came the razor. She shaved my head as smooth as a baby's behind. I in turn did the same to her head (minus the razor). Christine said it best, "I look like GI Jane and my husband looks like

Mr. Clean." Since then she's been able to smile a little more.

Kailey wanted to get her hair cut too, but ran away when she saw the scissors. She loves mom's head though, and told Christine, "Mommy's haircut beautiful," as she grabbed Chrissy's face and kisses her head. We have a downright angel in that one.

Chris went on-line to order some headpieces and a wig for the cold weather that appears to be quickly heading our way.

Sunday was another good day and Christine can't wait to get out of the house a little.

****

It was always good news when things started to get back to normal. An update from the doctor's office brought the news of Christine's blood counts getting back to normal after a chemotherapy treatment. I couldn't help but think how great everything seemed before having to go through a round of chemotherapy. Although Christine looked and felt fine, sometimes, as is the case with leukemia, things are not always as they seem. We knew that without the treatments, things would turn very bad for Christine.

Monday, October 6, 2003:

Christine received good news from the doctor today. Her blood-work shows that her immune system is back and her blood counts are rising steadily! She was extremely proud of the accomplishment and revels in the fact she was not readmitted to the hospital due to fever or other complications.

"Why is this an accomplishment?" you might ask.

Well, according to the medical staff, a large percentage (roughly 80%) of patients who receive this type of chemotherapy and are sent home without an immune system are readmitted to the hospital due to fever before their immune system comes back. Once you go back in, you stay in until your immune system returns because the fever means some type of infection is alive and running through the body.

The last thing the attending doctor said to Christine in the hospital before she came home was, "See you when you get a fever."

To which Christine responded, "Sorry, but I'm not getting a fever." (My feisty little lady!)

This was the 4th consecutive chemo round where Christine was not re-admitted despite the earlier statistic [if you count her initial treatments before relapse]. Some accomplishment if you ask me!

****

It's easy to get caught up in the hustle of moving from one procedure to the next. It's also a great feeling when things start to get back to normal. Despite the fewer visits to the doctor, the extra time to think about exactly what's going on can wear heavily on the mind, especially for the patient. My wife tried hard not to keep idle as she continued to "get better," but there's only so much you can do; and then you start to "think." It's healthy to "think," but it can become overwhelming. That's when the additional assistance of our support group, the Care for Christine Network, helped, especially when all the love and support was for her. Christine really benefited from those around us.

Thursday, October 9, 2003:

Christine's doctor appointment was cancelled for this past Tuesday because her blood work looked really good on Monday. That gave her the whole week to relax and enjoy not having to trek into the city.

Each day has its ups and downs though and Christine felt a little depressed on Tuesday. It's hard to blame her for feeling a mix of emotions as we approach the transplant date. She has the weight of the world on her shoulders and we're all doing our best in helping to keep some of the pressure off, but sometimes I can tell its wearing on her. HOWEVER! with every letter, card, message, e-mail, phone call, plate of food, cake (caramel chocolate), etc. that she receives, a piece of the world is held a little bit higher, and she knows that we're with her all the way.
I don't think you can all appreciate the magnitude of your support, and my words could not do it justice. Thanks.

****

It's always nice to hit a milestone, but in the case of a BMT there is such a long road to recovery that before long it's back to the grind of the doctor visits. You're very quickly reminded of your next steps. A strong will and unwavering determination are a must, and you need them to stay strong.

Friday, October 10, 2003:

Today's doctor appointment was rather routine, checking Christine's blood counts to make sure they're in line with normal measures. They looked good once again, and Christine is off until next Wednesday when she goes back to see her transplant doctor for a check-up.

Christine was told that she will undergo tests to register her baseline blood readings prior to going into transplant. They do this after every chemotherapy treatment to ensure they know a person's starting point for the next procedure.

As you all know from reading my updates, Christine is scheduled to go into the hospital for the transplant on Oct 27th, meaning we'll be in for Halloween.

****

Collecting information and doing research was a standard part of our journey, from Christine's initial diagnosis until well beyond her transplant. It was a way to ensure we were doing what was right for Christine, as well as to not get blindsided by what was to come. I tried to share whatever information I could with everyone around, everyone who cared, to ensure we were all on the same page whether physically by Christine's side or not. The following update was by far the most informative I had given to date and it would set the tone for Christine's battles to come. This information, in the right hands, would possibly save her life.

Wednesday, October 15, 2003:

Christine went through a number of tests today and she did very well. She also received a full run down of the BMT agenda. It was a lot of information to receive in one day, but it answered a lot of outstanding questions that we all had about the transplant.

Check below for a full explanation of the process in our own words. There are a lot of fine details for all of our friends and family to read about. I strongly recommend EVERYONE read the process so you know what to expect from Christine and our family for at least the next year. A year may sound like a long time, but once you consider the accomplishment, it's a drop in the bucket. Her Doctor said it nicely this morning, "The hardships in the short term are so you can reap the benefits in the long term."

Transplant Information:

Our original hospital date of October 27th has been moved slightly to November 3rd.

Christine will be in the hospital for roughly five to seven weeks once she's admitted. Hopefully, she will be out of the hospital for Christmas and refuses to think about a holiday season spent away from home, except for Thanksgiving. Thanksgiving will be a different story, although we will continue the tradition of playing Christmas carols after Santa Claus makes his appearance in the Thanksgiving Day parade, we will be spending it in the hospital.

During her stay in the hospital, Christine will be confined to her room, only leaving to take x-rays and go through other procedures. Although the visiting rules are not very strict in the hospital, for Christine's safety we are asking that only immediate family visit. Immediate family will be required to wash their hands thoroughly and wear a mask, gown and gloves when entering her room.

If anyone even thinks they may have a cold, or have been around anyone they know has had a cold, we ask that you use your best judgment and postpone your visit until you're absolutely certain. **Christine's life depends on it.**

Christine is scheduled to begin her procedures a day after being admitted to the hospital. Beginning November 4th Chrissy will receive radiation treatments for four consecutive days. The treatments will consist of approximately 20 minutes of radiation given three times a day. Her last day of radiation will be on November 7th.

On November 8th and November 9th Chrissy will begin receiving doses of chemotherapy. She will receive two different types of chemotherapy. One is a high dose chemo and the other a low dose chemo [referring to strength and intensity].

On November 10th through November 12th, Christine will finish her treatments with low dose chemotherapy only. The purpose of the radiation and chemotherapy will be to kill her existing immune system and her body's ability to create blood cells. The treatment will bring everything to such low levels that nothing will be able to grow back on its own.

November 13th will be an off day.

On November 14th, probably in the evening, Christine will receive the donor's bone marrow. It is usually given through an IV drip, very similar to the way she would receive a normal blood transfusion.

November 14th is considered Day Zero. Each day following the transplant date adds a number, so if I were to say "day 5," it refers to five days post-transplant.

From days one to fourteen Christine will experience some of the more common side effects of a BMT, mostly due to the radiation and chemotherapy. These include nausea, mouth and throat sores causing discomfort when eating solid foods, amongst others. Her immune system will be gone and she will be given antibiotics, antiviral medications, anti-fungal medications, and other medicines to help her fight off anything that could be dangerous to her.

At around day 14 the donor's bone marrow will have had enough time to set itself and begin to grow blood cells. Once Christine's new blood cells are being created and are at levels the doctors are happy with, she will be sent home.

Home is a much more sanitary place than the hospital, even with Christine in reverse isolation [every one of us visiting Christine's isolated room had to wear mask, gown, and gloves to avoid spreading germs]. Although Christine will be home, she will still be without an immune system for some time. She will have to visit the doctor for weekly checkups and check back into the hospital if she gets sick.

Christine will be without a full immune system for anywhere from 6 months to 2 years. This means she will need to take special care when being around other people, and will have to continue to limit the number of visitors she is able to see post-transplant. The reason for the lengthy period of time for the immune system to return is due to the T-cell depleted transplant Christine will be receiving.

T-cells are the part of the immune system [white blood cells] that fight off infection and disease, however these cells would also be the cause of a side effect known as "Graft vs. Host" (GVH) disease. This is a condition in which the T-cells in the bone marrow from the donor rejects Christine's body. By removing most of the T-cells in the blood, the probability of GVH disease and the extent of its seriousness are reduced. The caveat is a longer recovery time for the immune system.

The first three months post-transplant will be the most difficult part of the recovery period. Christine will have to take very good care of herself and so will we.

Once Christine hits day 100, the first crucial milestone, she will be able to go out to familiar restaurants and begin to enjoy more and more of what she's been missing by being confined. The farther she gets away from the transplant date the more of her life she'll be able to take back.

Every two months the doctor will run tests to see if Christine's blood is producing T-cells. When the T-cells are confirmed to be present, we will know Christine has a functioning immune system. Once the doctors are happy that Christine is through any long term side effects, and her body is producing infection and disease fighting cells, she'll get the thumbs up. Whether it takes Christine six months to regain her new immune system or two years, it will definitely have been worth the wait.

****

Keeping ourselves busy in between the tests and before the transplant was the objective leading up to the transplant date. We all tried to keep Christine doing what she loved to do. Throughout the updates I will mention understanding more about what life is truly all about, most of the time taking a step back and observing what was around us; looking at the obvious. We don't do that often enough when we "grow-up." It's not too late to realize it though. It's only a shame if you fail to realize it early enough to enjoy it; to have it matter in your life.

Friday, October 17, 2003:

We are in Rhode Island! We're having a nice relaxing time up here visiting my sister Tracy.

We did some shopping this evening and ate dinner out. Christine bought a bunch of things in The Christmas Tree Shop. I'm not sure what she bought, but she was smiling and I know it wasn't a Christmas tree. She's a lot like her mom that way. Those two love to shop.

Christine had a very long week with many tests throughout. Her latest test was a "muga" in which they injected radioactive isotopes into her bloodstream and monitored them as she rested. She then rode a stationary bike. I was in the room with my mother in-law when Christine was doing the test and I had an amazing "moment."

The test involves two big cameras that take pictures of Christine's blood-flow through her heart. The cameras can see the injected radio-isotope. The end-product is a picture by picture movie of Christine's beating heart. The "moment" came as I gazed at the computer screen in the test room; right there in front of me, was the picture of my wife's heart, beating; the heart that I love with all of my own; the reason for Christine's strength and passion.

I stared long and hard at the image as it pulsed at a steady pace on the screen. I can't express the feelings that rushed through my body at that moment. The feelings that made me want to run in and pick up Christine and hug her with all of my strength. I knew right there, more than ever, that she is going to be alright when the transplant and her recovery are completed. It's funny that as big as her heart was up on that screen, I know how much bigger it truly is.

****

Call it nervous energy but sometimes I just had to write. I was extremely nervous as Christine's BMT approached and there was really nothing I could do about it that didn't make me worry Christine would lose any kind of confidence she'd mustered preparing for what was to come. For her to be confident I knew I had to be. Not really knowing what to expect despite having been given the rundown of events, we braced for the countdown and tried to enjoy every last minute before the moment of truth.

Monday, October 27, 2003:

Christine has exactly one week from today before her BMT treatment begins. On November 3rd, Christine will go into the hospital to begin her regimen of radiation and chemotherapy. Shortly following the preparation treatments, she'll receive the donor's marrow.

Christine and I, along with her mom and dad, have spent a great deal of time going over the procedures with her doctors.

We spent a really nice weekend relaxing and doing some work around the house. We finished it off with a great turkey dinner at Christine's parents' house on Sunday. It was like an early Thanksgiving minus the stuffed mushrooms [one of Christine's favorites, but mushrooms were on the "restricted food list."]

Christine's hair is beginning to come back slightly despite the fact it will fall out again after the coming treatments. It looks to be coming back very blonde. It's funny that she went from blonde to brunette and now possibly back to blonde. After the transplant and after recuperation, it will be interesting to see what the final hair color will be.

Thanks to everyone for the continued support and prayers as we get closer to November 3rd. We can feel the love, support and the backing of all our friends and family. It makes it a little easier knowing we have all of you behind us. Christine has continued to read every message that comes in. She loves hearing from everyone.

****

The day finally came and one of my fears rang true. I came down with a cold. It would be the first time ever I was not able to be beside my wife and during her biggest challenge yet; radiation treatments. It was however a blessing to have our family so close to us to help. As I tried to get healthy so I could make my way back to her I knew she was in good hands.

During the ordeal, I did get to spend extra time with my daughter. I never told anyone, but the nights with Kailey and I home alone sent a chill down my spine. I tried to avoid negative thoughts. I cried a lot during those nights after Kailey fell asleep. I prayed nightly that this was a temporary thing. I prayed 'two' would one day be 'three' again within the walls of our home. It just had to.

Tuesday, November 4, 2003:

Christine was admitted to the hospital yesterday at approximately 4:30PM. There was a slight delay due to some issues with medical coverage. We were able to work it out however with some great work by key individuals in my company, Christine's doctor, the insurance company doctor who reviewed the appeal, and a number of our friends who were able to point us in the right direction.

I never in my life want to experience my wife having to say goodbye to our daughter ever again. It has to be the single most heartbreaking moment ever. I can't even write anymore about it right now. I just can't.

Once Christine was settled into the hospital she sounded great. She was ready for the battle and her spirits were high.

Christine began her radiation treatments today at noon. She had another session at 6pm and will have three sessions a day for the next three days. Unfortunately, the radiation comes with nausea, something that has been the single most consistent issue with Chrissy throughout all of her treatments. Hopefully, the doctors can find the right medication that makes her feel well. This evening Christine sounded a little out of it over the phone, most likely due to being worn out from the radiation and medication.

I am currently unable to stay with Christine in the hospital due to a cold I have had for the last 5 days. I'm hoping to get rid of it as soon as possible. I'm loading up on vitamin C. I'm also drinking lots of liquids and trying my darndest to get back to her. Christine's Mom is spending the nights with her while I cannot. I have been spending time at home recuperating.

Tonight it's just Kailey and I. Kailey made mommy a stuffed construction paper fish. We named her "Kailey's Fish of Anti-Nausea" and Christine will receive it in the morning. Hopefully it helps a little, or at least brings a smile to her face.

We were able to get webcams working and Christine has a laptop in the hospital. The Tech team over at MSKCC set her up with an internet connection and she'll be able to surf the net and do some Christmas shopping once she's feeling up to it.

We'll test the video conferencing very soon so she can see Kailey at home whenever she wants. If the connection to the hospital works, it will be a BIG step toward more smiles.

Keep praying....we love you all.

****

The intensive radiation wasn't an easy thing for Christine to endure but the side effects were something that would become regular occurrences through the coming months. Still sick, I spoke with Christine often as I tried more and more to rid myself of the cold. Visiting Christine at this point could have been a bad thing for all of us. One wrong move could jeopardize everything.

<u>Saturday, November 8, 2003:</u>

Christine is now complete with her 4 days and 11 sessions of radiation. She was as much on a puking schedule as she was on a treatment schedule. Christine was a little embarrassed when she had to stop the technicians from administering the radiation to vomit, but she said it looked like they were used to it (with a chuckle).

The radiation was a little tougher on her than she expected, but she got through it. She starts her chemotherapy today and will also receive a special serum treatment derived from horses. The serum is administered over 8 hours and is an immunosuppressive treatment to help ensure she does not reject the donor's bone marrow. The chemotherapy will be administered after that and will be given over a 2-4 hour period.

She will receive this chemo for two days. It is the lighter of the two. On chemo day 3 & 4, Christine will receive a chemotherapy called Cytoxan which will be the roughest part of the treatment so far. This is a deviation from the original plan, but it has more of an anti-leukemic effect than the previously planned chemo.

Christine is fighting strong and looks so cute lying in bed over the webcam, even if she is suffering a bit.

I am still sick but getting better day by day. My doctor said I have to wait it out because it's a cold and there's very little I can do to treat it. I have been taking cold medicine and vitamin C, vegetable and fruit juices, Cold-eeze, multi-vitamins, and soup to get rid of this thing. Hopefully it goes away soon. Thanks to many of you for your care, efforts, and supplies in trying to get me well enough to get back in the fight with my wife.

****

Each day, one small step at a time; baby steps were progress. Finally getting into the hospital with my wife was a highlight I wouldn't soon forget. Christine was most definitely in the middle of the war when I was finally able to visit her in the hospital.

The many requests for blood donations to family, friends and colleagues were paying off. Christine needed dozens of blood transfusions during this time and the web site and updates had already paid for themselves many times over in love, support and blood donations. I had a small fear that Christine was in her current condition and her fate rested in the hands (or stem cells) of a complete stranger; our silent hero who we knew nothing about. I prayed that he would come through for us. If he backed out now I feared all would be lost.

<u>**Monday, November 10, 2003:**</u>

I was finally able to visit Christine today and although I came home this evening as a precaution, I can't tell you how amazing it was to finally see her after a full week. Christine is an absolute inspiration and I hold my head high with pride when saying she's my wife. She is a true warrior and has the courage of a champion. I love her so much.

CHRISTINE IS FINISHED WITH HER RADIATION AND CHEMO! She finished her last bag of chemo today and although the road has been tough so far, she is doing wonderfully. I have never seen such raw determination in anyone.

Christine's last 8 days have been anything but comfortable and that's putting it lightly. Just to give you a brief glimpse into what she's going through, today I witnessed Christine vomit at least 6 times, and at times she was throwing up blood.

She has not been able to eat for about 6 days and they've been giving her plenty of fluid through IV to make up for it as much as possible. Christine has had numerous red blood and platelet transfusions. THANKS to EVERYONE who was able to donate so far. It's going to good use.

Christine's BMT has been pushed up from Friday to Thursday due to the stem cells being available a day earlier than expected.

The transplant will consist of a vial of "baby blood cells" [stem cells an equivalent of bone marrow] being pushed into Christine's blood stream through the port that was surgically put into her chest. It's a T-Cell depleted transplant and it should be a quick procedure. Some of you [including me] thought the transplant might consist of major surgery. Thank goodness this isn't the case.

Although the chemo and radiation are finished, Chris still has a long road to go; about 4-7 more weeks in the hospital and a whole lot of recovery after that. Please keep the messages and prayers coming

****

Preparation for receiving the stem cells was kicking Christine's butt. In the immortal words of Vince Lombardi though, "It's not whether you get knocked down; it's whether you get back up that counts." Christine was living his words day in and day out. Each and every time she got knocked down she was up again. Vince would have been proud, especially since Christine's big moment was quickly arriving. It's always nice to get a little emotional push along the way as well. Enter our hero.

Day-0, Thursday, November 13, 2003 (afternoon):

Tonight's the night! Chrissy is all set to receive the BMT this evening at approximately 9PM! It was recently moved from 8PM simply due to how long it took the lab to work on the T-cell depletion.

Although there will be an extended time for recovery, we are all excited and happy to get through Day-0 and begin the positive count to recovery. Tomorrow starts day-1. Keep the prayers coming along with the messages. Thanks to everyone for the blood donations, prayers and support. Our families are so grateful for all you have done and all you continue to do.

An Amazing Message! The nurse practitioner came into the room today at about 5:30PM. She was smiling and said she had a surprise.

"A surprise?!" we asked.

In her possession was a hand written letter from Christine's donor. It was a very emotional moment for us all, as we read the words written from our new faceless and nameless friend. His words were sweet and sincere. A message brought on angel's wings.

Good luck and God bless my wife as the transplant approaches. We love you Chrissy!

****

The road to recovery was about to begin and we were all very excited. I felt like this was such a special occasion that it should have been on the big screen in time square, or on national television. Since those weren't options I went for the next best thing. We needed our daughter and others close to us to see Christine's life being saved. The countdown is over and the count-up begins here. Starting at Day-0, the daily count would be an important indicator for milestones and a guideline for her recovery.

Day 0, Thursday, November 13, 2003 (evening):

Christine's transplant began at 9:35PM and ended at 9:52PM on November 13.

Christine now has a second birthday. The nurse said every year, for this birthday, she gets jewels. It's hard to disagree.

I broadcast the transplant over the internet to my mom and dad, our daughter Kailey, and my sister Tracy in Rhode Island. Christine's mom, dad and I were in the hospital room with her for the procedure with the doctor, a fellow, and the nurse and we all shared the miraculous moment together, just as it should be.

Today is considered Christine's second birthday; mark November 13, 2003 on your calendars. It's the first day of the rest of Christine's new life.

Happy Birthday Christine!

****

At the time Christine received the transplant, the push of the donor's stem cells into her body, the full effects of the radiation and chemotherapy had not yet fully shown their ugly face. She was beginning to feel the effects, but unfortunately the worst of it was still to come. Christine's journey was going to get a lot tougher before it got better.

Day 2, Saturday, November 15, 2003:

Christine's fight continues as she has experienced increased pain and discomfort due to the effects of the chemo and radiation. The pain should continue until her blood counts begin to come back to normal levels. That may take up to a month, but can happen earlier. The medical staff has increased her pain medication to help make her as comfortable as possible.

I read the [support network] messages to Christine every day and she sometimes logs in and checks them herself. She began Christmas shopping over the web yesterday and has made a few purchases. It's funny to see her and her mom sitting at the computer shopping away. I know it helps to take her mind off the pain a little and the time passes by a little more quickly for her. Any relief she finds only lasts for a short time though and then she needs to lie down.

****

Baby steps are the way of recovery. Each and every minor achievement is a blessing. In building back this house, each and every brick deserves a celebration and sometimes a small show of anything positive is more than anyone would have hoped for in a given day. I spend some time in the following update going into more detail about the side effects she's experiencing.

Day 7, Thursday, November 20, 2003:

We've Got Counts! After one full week of low blood counts, and a white blood count of 0, the first sign of Christine's white blood growing back showed itself today! After exactly 7 days of nothing, the white blood counts came back with a reading of .1. Yes, it's only point one, but it's not zero. That means the bone marrow may have found its home and is starting to make blood again.

According to the doctor, the bone marrow or stem cells are so smart that they actually find their way to the correct location in the body within 24 hours of the transplant. That's why, directly after the transplant, they do not take any blood from the patient. They wait 24 hours to avoid pulling any of the bone marrow out of the body before it finds its way to its new home.

A Tough Road So Far

Christine has spent the last 2 weeks in a tough battle against the side effects of the radiation and chemotherapy. The mornings are predominantly the worst time of day, with vomiting and pain keeping her very uncomfortable, however, her fight to stay strong and keep her chin up sometimes has her smiling through the pain by noon. Chrissy has not eaten for roughly two and a half weeks. She is now finding nourishment in the form of an IV drip called TPN, or Total Parenteral Nutrition. It's a big yellow bag of fluid containing all the vitamins and minerals she needs to stay healthy. Christine currently can't eat because of the sores that have formed in her mouth and throat. The sores are caused by the radiation and chemotherapy which have the most dramatic effect on fast growing cells in the body. These include the cells found in the mouth, throat, stomach, and hair amongst others.

Despite the TPN, Christine is hungry and can't wait to eat SHRIMP! She has been craving it every day and can't wait for it not to burn when she eats something. She was finally able to take medication via mouth without throwing it up today; a small but very significant form of progress.

Getting Up and About

Christine has continued to keep herself as busy as possible until exhaustion forces her to lie down. She has spent hours on the computer shopping, reading messages from all of you, or playing solitaire. She has also decorated a few Christmas ornaments, painting 3 Christmas balls given to her by the recreation area on the 15th floor here at MSKCC. They are absolutely fantastic on 15. They went out of their way to put some crafty things together for Christine to do. It's an amazing amazing amazing program for the patients here at the hospital. They even have a pool table up there.

Keeping in Touch

Thanks to everyone who has sent messages to Christine. We'd like to send a special thanks to our most frequent poster, Christine's cousin Jessica. All cards that were sent to our home were brought to her and are hanging on her hospital wall.

****

Ups and downs were a big part of the recovery process throughout. I quickly learned that what the doctors and nurses expected was based on experience and not always through medical science. We had to keep reminding ourselves that we were in the middle of the worst part of the early side effects and patience was our ally. One good thing was that as new side effects emerged, others seemed to go away, at least temporarily.

Day 8, Friday, November 21, 2003:

Today Christine's white counts were back down at zero. The medical staff told us this would happen and we are not surprised as point one (.1) wasn't a very high count to begin with. At least we know the counts are doing something and that she has what looks like working bone marrow. It's just a matter of time before they come back even higher. (Insert prayers here.)

Christine is feeling a little tired today and mouth sores seemed to spring up overnight. She had been suffering more from throat sores, but it seems the mouth sores were just delayed a little. Hopefully they heal quickly, but we need white counts for that to happen.

The sores are getting so bad that it's difficult for Christine to talk, so she's been trying to avoid it whenever possible. She actually told me, "You better start anticipating what I'm going to say."

I nodded my head, "Yes dear."

It's now going on two and a half weeks since the last time she's eaten and they still have the TPN[nutritional supplement] dripping around the clock. They have even given her a white substance to compensate for fat intake. They're dripping lipids into her body. They have this whole nutrition thing covered, even if it is through tubes.

Christine has been able to get up and roam about her room at different times during the day. She gets tired quickly however and then has to lie down and rest. We're hoping the white counts start to make their way back in larger numbers soon.

Because Christine's mouth sores and an excess mucus condition seemed to get worse today, the doctors are going to start her on a drug called Neupogen (GCSF or G). G is a drug invented by Sloan Kettering which acts as a catalyst for the body to produce white blood cells. This will help Christine's body in producing white blood cells more quickly and hopefully help speed up her healing process.

The sores and excess mucus will start to go away when her white counts get to about point eight (.8) or higher.

Christine received GCSF after every chemotherapy treatment prior to the transplant. She gave herself a shot in the stomach area for about 14 consecutive days after each chemo round. This time around the nurses will give it to her.

The good news is Christine hasn't thrown up at all today! It's "funny" when that's the highlight of your day, but baby steps are what make us happy.

****

It's tough measuring what 'bad' means when you're going through something for the first time and only have the experience and words of others to set your expectations. When you expect bad things and they're even worse than expected it most definitely wears on you. When this happened it was when we needed each other the most. Christine needed us to help her keep up the fight. She needed Kailey's picture, our words of encouragement, and the letters and notes from all those around us to get over the hump. Sometimes it seems we're put to the test and brought right to the verge of breaking before the clouds part and sun peeks through. On day-9 the clouds were definitely out.

<u>Day 9, Saturday, November 22, 2003:</u>

What a difference a day can make. The only good news about today was Christine's white counts were at point three (.3) but the doctors and nurses said they'll probably go down to zero again.

This had to be the worst day yet. Christine woke up feeling absolutely horrible. The mouth and throat sores were the most painful they've been so far. The doctors upped the amount of pain medication Christine is receiving in an attempt to make her more comfortable.

Christine hasn't had a fever since she first came into the hospital, which is great, but the pain is unbearable without the medication.

When it rains it pours of course. She has been throwing up since we woke up this morning. I lost count of how many times she vomited when we got to 10.

I felt so badly for her today. I spent some time rubbing her feet and her back, which became very sore from the stress of throwing up. The thing that helped most though seemed to be a drug called Ativan. Ativan is for anxiety, which also usually helps her with nausea, sleeping, and some of the pain. The relief still wasn't as much as she seemed to need and the vomiting continued.

Christine came close to losing it today. Besides the pain, sores and vomiting, there's one more thing that decided to show its ugly face.

We've heard a lot about mouth sores and excess mucus and their inevitability; however, we didn't actually realize that with the mouth sores comes an actual shedding of the skin in the mouth and throat. It really all comes off, and it's not a thin layer of skin either.

At some point during the early evening, a strip of skin began to peel away from the roof of Christine's mouth. She was immediately instructed not to pull or tug at the skin because pulling it could potentially cause it to "bleed like a geyser," an actual quote from the nurse. So the skin began to peel throughout her mouth and she couldn't do a thing about it except rinse her mouth with a special solution and wait for the dead skin to fall off by itself. The solution contains a topical drug called Lidocaine and makes the mouth pain easier to bear.

All in all this had to be the most frustrating and painful day so far. It's so hard to see her go through this. I hope and pray it gets better tomorrow.

****

Despite 'Day 9' and like *The Little Train Who Could*, Christine made it to the peak of the hill pulling a very heavy load. All the while 'We knew she could.'

Day 10, Sunday, November 23, 2003:

As I said in Day 9's update, "It's amazing how much of a difference a day can make."

I woke up this morning and looked across to see Christine sitting up in bed. I ask her if things were alright and she said, "Yes."

I could tell by the way she answered and the tone of her voice that things were starting to get better. She was more awake than she had been the entire day before and her reaction to my question was 10 times better. I popped up and stared over at her and she smiled. Two pieces of skin that were bothering her in her mouth had fallen off as she did one of the many rinses she does daily. There were still more in there, but she was even starting to look much better.

The best news of the day was Christine's white blood count reported back at 3! That's not point three (.3), but THREE. Ten times the count from Day 9. The doctor came in and commented on how nice the blood counts were looking. Christine's pain was a little better and she only vomited twice throughout the day, a big improvement over the day before. We were so happy and can only pray that the counts continue to move upward.

****

We hadn't really mentioned home yet in the updates, simply focusing on Christine getting better. Like a team that's 3 games down in the World Series we needed to focus on one game at a time before thinking of being world champs. As Christine's white blood counts continued to rise however, the realization hit that she was getting closer and closer to home. It was absolutely amazing how much better she became after the white blood cells circulated through her body and started healing all the sores that had come out uncontested. We started to get a glimpse at what her new blood was capable of. We liked what we saw. Where had this blood come from!?

Day 11, Monday, November 24, 2003:

Christine's white counts were 19.8 today!!! The GCSF [a drug that helps stimulate white blood cell growth] coupled with the bone marrow, started to generate white counts earlier than expected and the counts are well above normal.

The objective was to have the bone marrow produce a blood count of approximately 20(the norm is between 4 and 10.) Then they would stop the GCSF shots and see where the white counts leveled off. We expected this to be at or after Day 12 and we're already there at Day 11!

We were so happy today to have her counts on the rise. They stopped the GCSF shots today.

Christine was in better condition today. Almost all of the dead skin and sores in her mouth are gone. Her throat and mouth are feeling much better.

She took her first bite of something to eat at exactly 4:27PM tonight; 2 spoonfuls of Dannon Whipped Yogurt!

She's a real trooper and I cannot tell you how happy we are that she seems to have turned a corner past the most physically painful part of the chemotherapy and radiation side effects. We know that we're far from out of the woods, but we continue to remain positive. We look forward to Christine eating more and eventually making her way home. If her white counts stay high, the doctors will start reducing some of her medication.

Once Christine's body starts creating T-Cells in her white blood cells, she'll be closer to having a full immune system. The catch is she'll have the equivalent immune system of a newborn and will probably have to go through immunizations again. We have a little while before we have to think about that though.

We continue to pray that her white counts stay where they need to be and her red and platelet counts make their way back to normal as well.

****

Spending holidays in the hospital were something we were getting used to. This year our main objective was to get Christine home for Christmas. Thanksgiving was to be spent in the hospital, but it was special none the less. We had a lot to be thankful for this year. Some people might not have looked at it that way. As far as we were concerned, Christine was on what looked like the road to recovery and we were surrounded by people who supported us on the inside and out. This Thanksgiving we received a special delivery from a good friend and her family.

Day 14, Thursday, November 27, 2003,

Thanksgiving Day:

Christine's progress has been slow but steady. She has been able to eat chicken broth and some noodles, but didn't have as much luck with the turkey.

Her white blood counts have started their decline back toward normal levels and although we have a bit to go, she's moving in the right direction. The white counts are currently 44.6. Normal levels are between 4 and 11. This is normal for her procedure and we'll have to wait to see where they level off.

Christine remains in good spirits despite the fatigue, and she was even able to ride the stationary bike for 15 minutes yesterday and today for some exercise.

Because her white counts have remained elevated the doctors have removed her antibiotics and most of the other medications protecting her while her immunity was 0. Her mouth sores are totally healed and the biggest issue is that her stomach is not used to solid food. She will probably have to stay with a fluid diet until she can handle the solids and the vomiting subsides. In the meantime the doctors still have her on TPN to make sure she's getting what she needs nutritionally.

Big Thanksgiving Surprise!

I stayed home with Kailey on Wednesday night and came back into the hospital at about 3:30PM today to spend the rest of the day with Christine, my brother in-law, and my mother and father in-law. While home, Kailey and I watched the Thanksgiving Day parade along with Christine over the webcam.

As tradition goes in our family, we all danced around to Christmas songs once Santa came to town at the end of the parade; Christine danced a little from her hospital bed. Kailey was so excited to see Santa that she cheered, jumped up and down and clapped with a huge smile on her face. Shortly after our third Christmas song, Kailey fell asleep in my arms as we danced. It's the most amazing feeling to have your daughter fall asleep on your shoulder. It goes hand in hand with her telling you she loves you, and an unexpected kiss on the cheek.

After returning to the hospital in the afternoon, we all received a fantastic surprise. At 5:00PM we were treated to a special delivery from our friends in Astoria, Queens...Thanksgiving dinner! I will not mention names here, but I would like this friend and her family to know that their generosity will forever be remembered.

We all ate like kings and queens and although this might sound cruel since she can't really eat yet, Christine savored the smell after trying to put away some of the turkey unsuccessfully. Once again, thanks so much for this wonderful Thanksgiving surprise! It was appreciated more than words can say.

To all our friends and family,

As the Thanksgiving Day comes to a close, the day would not be complete, for us, without wishing all of you a warm and loving "Happy Thanksgiving." Your love, support, and prayers, your jokes, messages and stories have all helped to make our road to this Thanksgiving that much easier, and have helped us to remain that much stronger. We love you and thank you from the bottom of our hearts.

All our love,
The Wonica and the Dragula families
Happy Thanksgiving!

****

I was beside myself with love and happiness on this Thanksgiving Day. I needed to vent and share it with those around me. I sat down and spilled my heart into a letter. I didn't write it for anyone in particular and yet I wrote it for anyone and everyone. I was blessed and I knew it. On that Thanksgiving Day, I was on top of the world.

<u>My Thanksgiving Note...</u>

As it gets closer to midnight and the end of Thanksgiving 2003, I reflect on my life and the things that have gone on around me and my family. I look at the obstacles and the trials we have faced and are currently working to overcome.

Our troubles have been great and much more than I ever thought I would experience by the age of 29. I look upon these times though and I smile. I smile, because I am thankful.

I am thankful for my wife and the strength we have as a married couple; her smile, her love, and her beauty inside and out; the way she looks at me when I'm acting silly, and the way she looks at me when she knows I'm serious; the way she listens.

I am thankful for her organizational skills :-) and the way she makes me stronger and challenges me to be the best I can be. I am thankful for our life together.

I am thankful for the beautiful daughter she has given me, the newest reason for us to keep up our fight; for the time I get to spend with Kailey and the love she shows me; for her unexpected kisses, the way she dances to her favorite songs, and the words she tries to say but can't (yet). I am thankful she loves to run and can swing a bat and throw a ball. I am thankful she looks like Christine. I am thankful for her morning calls of "Dad, come here!" when she wakes up. I am thankful for each and every morning she tells me she wants waffles for breakfast and for each and every time she falls asleep in my arms.

I am thankful for the home we have built and the family and friends who helped along the way; for the family we are and always will be; for my mother and father and my sisters and brother; for my grandparents, aunts, uncles, cousins and all my family.

I am thankful for Christine's mom and dad, her brother, Nana and grandma and all her aunts, uncles, cousins and the rest of her family; for all our friends, colleagues, teammates and former teammates; for the love and support you have all shown, and the prayers we have received and continue to receive.

I am thankful for the help of our parents, the help of our parents and the help of our parents; oh, and the help of our parents. Did I mention the help of our parents? (You get the picture.)

Same as the previous paragraph but substitute 'help' with 'love.'

I am especially thankful for complete strangers who donate the gift of life, more specifically the unknown stem cell donor who has given Christine new life; our own personal living angel.

I am thankful for God and his angels, and for blessings and prayer. I am thankful for the faith to believe, and for the will to stay on the right path. I am thankful for people with big hearts, O+ blood, and a lot of platelets; for the ears of those who care; and the support of angels on earth.

I am thankful for The Leukemia & Lymphoma Society[2], for the American Cancer Society, for Light The Night, and for Team in Training.

---

[2] The Leukemia & Lymphoma Society can be found on the internet at http://lls.org

I am thankful for friends who run marathons and participate in fundraising walks to fight this and other diseases. I am thankful for doctors and nurses and for MSKCC. I am thankful for medical benefits and when issues with insurance companies work out in the end.

I am thankful for letters to my wife from 6th grade classes in IS 24 room 608 [my cousin Alexis' class].

I am thankful for you.

I am thankful for so much...for so much.

I'm sure my list is different than yours. I would apologize for its length, but it's long for a reason. The fact is it could have been a whole lot longer. We all have our own things that we're thankful for, but the thing that is most important, is that we all have a list.

Christine says I'm an eternal optimist. Take another look above. How can I not be?

All my love, God bless, and Happy Thanksgiving,

Tommy

****

Getting better and better was the thing we liked to see. Sloan Kettering was an amazing hospital with a staff I'd put at the top of any list. The doctors and nurses were absolutely incredible in helping her recover. When you're in the same room with limited visitors for almost a straight month it starts to feel a lot like a prison and 'stir crazy' becomes part of your day to day reality. The better Christine felt the more she thought about getting home to our little girl; the more she wanted to hold Kailey in her arms.

Day 18, Monday, December 1, 2003:

Christine has continued to make progress over the last couple of days. Her white counts are coming down within the normal range of 4-11 and should level off in the next few days.

Her red blood counts and platelets have started to rise on their own. The doctors say there's a chance the counts may dip once again and then rise. It's primarily day by day as Christine improves.

Chrissy is looking better and better each day. She is up and about and as I type this she is sitting in a chair reading a book on "how to go home after a stem cell transplant." You can see where her mind is.

She has been able to eat a little bit more each day, although it is still very little. Christine has been able to drink Carnation instant breakfast; chocolate, with lactaide. She's also been nibbling on bread with beef broth her mom bought from the store.

Christine will begin writing down what she eats today for the staff to begin tracking her calories. She needs to eat and drink at least 1000 a day before they'll let her go home. Christine is working on it and can't wait.

Missing Home

As Christine gets better her longing to be home with our daughter gets worse. She has cried each of the last 4 days and I'm sure there will be more tears before she gets out of here. It has been difficult for her and all I can say is the more tears there are the better she feels. We keep reinforcing the fact that her stay here is temporary and that she will be home very soon.

We most likely have less than 2 weeks left in the hospital. She's so close she can taste it, which at this point tastes a lot better than the Carnation Instant Breakfasts.

****

As Christine continued to get stronger and take more steps toward going home, so many other little things would pop up that we hadn't considered. Who knew Christine would have such a hard time physically holding down solid foods for so long? Who knew that her body would build a slight dependence on the pain killers? Every little detail told its own story and each day we listened. This was also the time our support network started to show an even stronger commitment to our cause. One friend in particular decided he was going to run a marathon in Christine's honor as well as fight blood cancers at the same time. There would be more family and friends doing the same in the future, many doing things in honor of Christine. Everyday held a new lesson for us in both humility and inspiration. Day 19 was no different.

Day 19, Tuesday, December 2, 2003:

Funny thing about pain medication is that when your body is used to getting it for so long it tends to really want it. The 'fidgets' Christine currently has, are primarily due the pain medicine she is being weaned off because she no longer needs. It's driving her mad but they should only last for a day.

Another "funny" thing is she still has the fidgets when she sleeps. I don't know how that's possible, but I can't help but smile as she curses the feeling that makes her arms and legs just want to keep on moving. More importantly, they stopped her pain medication all together today. They had started to wean her gradually because of how serious opiate withdrawal can be. It could have been the reason for her puking episodes a few days ago. This is yet another difficult time, but very good news.

Christine hasn't puked in three days and was able to finish a WHOLE shake this morning and drank parts of shakes during the day. A WHOLE SHAKE PLUS!! She's hopefully on her way to real food soon and drinking the entire Carnation Breakfast shake was a huge milestone.

They have now started to also wean her off the TPN by giving it to her in cyclical fashion. That means continuously for 18 hours instead of 24, and then less and less and less and less, until she's down to no TPN at all. Something tells me Chrissy will miss that big yellow bag of flowing nutrients...NOT!

Her red blood counts broke 10 yesterday, coming back on their own. Normal is between 11 and 14.

Her platelets steadily rose for the fifth day in a row to 89. Normal is between 160 and 400, but these are usually the last blood cell type to return and Christine's are coming back very nicely.

Christine's white count was down to 11.3 yesterday. It will hopefully level off somewhere between the norm of 4 and 11. She's eagerly awaiting the call to the 'bullpen', "You're needed at home, start warming up." [Christine was a softball player in college and had received a full scholarship to LIU as a windmill pitcher so the analogy was fitting]. Soon, very soon. She wants to go home.

Tomorrow I'll try and run through some of the things Chrissy will be able to do when she gets home and what she cannot do. I'll tell you right now, I didn't like the smile on Christine's face when they said she can't cook or clean for a very long time. She was looking at me with eyes that said, "Now you're gunna get it!" Help…momma! Kidding of course, we just need to get her home.

My buddy Steve is running a marathon in Christine's honor, as part of the Leukemia & Lymphoma Society's Team in Training program. Details are on his website: http://SteveTornello.com [Steve's site now contains examples of his creative work – check it out if you have time!]

Enlightenment

Christine had some great words of advice today from her cousin Jessica. Christine needed this perspective more than ever as she's been missing Kailey something awful. The words were simple yet beautiful. These aren't her exact words, and I hope I can do them justice, so here it goes:

"Christine, you are lucky to have been given such an amazing gift. When this is all over, and you are home and as healthy as can be, you will have the gift of being able to look at life and all the things around you through eyes different than everyone else's.

You'll have a vision and insight into all the amazing things around you and you'll notice what most people take for granted every day. When you taste a piece of chocolate cake it will be the best piece of cake in the world; and when you smell a flower in the garden it will be the most precious smelling flower you've ever smelled, each and every time.

Walks in the park will be more than just a day out, time with loved one's more than just hanging around. Each and every moment will be cherished and hold special meaning that only you can understand."

Christine wiped a tear or two and realized how right Jessie was, how true her words actually were, and she smiled. Thanks Jess.

****

As the excitement built for Christine's homecoming and the worst short term dangers of the transplant seemed to be behind us I started to write a little more in each update. I continued to use the online journal as a source of therapy. I continued to use my writing as a way to give people a glimpse into our life at the time of recovery. I felt the Care for Christine supporters needed to know the impact of their continued support. Christine needed the continued positive energy the "Care for Christine Updates" generated. With all the excitement and focus on Christine however, we never forgot our little lady at home. Kailey was just 2 years old now and was fully aware that mommy hadn't been home for a long time. I was lucky enough to have been able to go home and stay with her occasionally and bring some normalcy to her life, and we were lucky my parents were able to keep her in our home almost every night so she knew she was safe while mommy and daddy weren't around. Regardless, Christine not able to be with Kailey was simply heart breaking. As the ground rules for homecoming were laid out, getting back to Kailey was at the top of the list.

Day 21, Friday, December 5, 2003:

We are on the tail end of day 21! 21 days since Christine's second birthday. She has been through a lot since the day we broadcast Chrissy receiving her new blood over the internet to our living room on Quinlan Ave.

She went through over 4 weeks of not eating, countless vomiting episodes, pain, sleepless nights, stress, anxiety, mouth sores, throat sores, stomach sores, peeling skin, back pain, etc... I am extremely pleased to write that Christine is doing wonderfully! She has progressed very nicely in her recovery and doing extremely well for someone having gone through a bone marrow transplant.

Christine's mouth and throat sores are all gone and eating is getting easier. She has been trying very hard to eat as much as she can tolerate because it'll take at least 1000 calories a day to get her home. She is just about there.

Christine's foods of choice have been canned peaches, pears, and Chocolate Carnation Instant Breakfast with Lactaid. As of this morning she tried dairy products for the first time in a while. The attempts seemed successful and tonight Christine had her share of Chocolate Carnation Instant Breakfast with Whole Milk and Vanilla Ice Cream!!! This was a big step for someone whose only food was a yellow syrupy fluid through a medi-port just a few days ago.

More good news! Because Christine has been eating so well, they skipped "cycling" off the TPN and stopped it all together. She is a woman on a mission!

Morning Check-ups

Each morning Christine's team of doctors comes into the room at about 10AM. They give her their review and give her a check-up. It's easy to see that they are very pleased with her progress.

Discussions have begun as to when she can come home. We're keeping our fingers crossed that it will be sooner, rather than later. She prays almost constantly that the time passes quickly so she can go home to see our daughter.

Kailey is missing mommy a lot too. She asks about Christine daily and only knows that "mommy will be home soon." "Soon" for a 2 year old can be an eternity.

Kailey picked up an advertisement the other day. It had a picture of a model who looked like Christine. Kailey picked up the ad with a big smile and excitement, kissed it and said, "Oh mommy." My mom was watching Kailey at the time and almost cried.

I explained to Kailey just this morning that mommy was doing well and her "boo boo" was getting a lot better. She cheered, jumped up and down and clapped her hands. "Soon" can't come quickly enough.

Due to the transplant, Christine is at an increased risk for a post-transplant disease called Epstein Barr Virus-related Lymphoproliferative Disorder, or EBV Lymphoma.

According to some research it looks like the likelihood of her getting this disorder is roughly 2%.

There is a preventative medicine called Rituximab (Rituxan), which may help prevent this EBV-Lymphoma. We will discuss this preventative medicine with a specialist in the morning. We want to make sure we have all our facts straight before we make a decision.

Coming Home: Rules and Regulations

I think it's safe to say that Christine will be coming home in the next week or so. When she does, there will be some strict rules she will have to follow in order to protect her from getting sick.

Since she will have a compromised immune system for some time, she will be diligent in following these rules. Trust me, Christine's diligence is 10,000 times my own, so you can bet she'll be on the ball with these rules.

<u>Here is the short list:</u>

1.   She can go outside in the yard and around the neighborhood without a mask

2. She can stay around all immediate family without anyone having to wear a mask as long as no one is sick or has been exposed to someone who is sick

3. She cannot cook or clean

4. She cannot garden

5. All plants and flowers must be moved out of the house

6. No Pets (our bird Amu must leave)

7. Due to the extra bad cold and flu season, Christine will not be receiving visitors AT ALL other than immediate family. It's for her safety. We'll let you know when this changes. We can't wait for this one to change!

8. Please do not send flowers because we will not be able to let them into the house.

9. Weekly Dr. visits will be required to ensure Christine's progress is monitored.

10. Chrissy will have to wait a little while for her first VERY VERY stiff drink. She deserves one though.

I think there may be more, but that's what I can remember for now. Number seven (7) is probably most important since I know a lot of you have been dying to see Chrissy. In the grand scheme of Christine's long life to be lived, just a little longer everyone....just a little longer.

Additional Notes

As I write this, Christine is sleeping by my side. I don't think I've seen Christine sleep this peacefully in a very long time. It's nice to see.

Christine thanked me tonight. She cried and thanked me for all I am doing for her and all I have done. I almost felt guilty. She told me that she couldn't do anything in the world to repay me. I have a few suggestions on how she can repay me:

1 Don't ever give up

2. Fight Fight Fight

3. Get well soon

For these things, there's nothing I can ever do, or anything I have ever done that can thank her enough for all she has given me. Yep, tonight Christine cried and thanked me for all I am doing for her and all I have done. I kissed her on the forehead and said,

"You're welcome." Sometimes that's just all you can do.

****

This update was the shortest but so very very exciting!

Day 25, December 8, 2003:

Christine is coming home today!!!

****

No background needed for the following update. This one speaks for itself as one of the most amazing.

Day 34, Wednesday, December 17, 2003:

I know, I know. Where have the updates been? I do apologize for the lack of information lately.

At first it was because what took place when Christine came home will be hard to explain. Words will not come close to the magic we experienced. Later on, I couldn't write because I was much too tired by the time midnight rolled around. That's when I usually write.

I was able to catch up on some sleep last weekend, so here it goes, my attempt at describing Chrissy's homecoming.

Christine's Update:

It has been one full week since Christine was released from the hospital and made her way home. She has continued her recovery and continues to do well.

It was a day of mixed emotions when Christine came home. She was so happy and excited to be getting out of the hospital, but at the same time she was nervous and frightened at what she'd experience living away from the medical attention she'd been receiving.

She was released on Dec 8th at about 2:45PM. We made it home by 3:30PM and my mom, dad, and Kailey were in the house as we pulled onto our block and pulled into our driveway on Quinlan Avenue.

Kailey had not seen Christine in person for exactly five weeks from the day Christine was admitted. She had stayed with my parents at our house for the duration. Kailey was still in her own environment, but she hadn't seen her Mom.

How would she react when Christine walked up to the house to say hello for the first time in what felt like a century?

Would she be angry at her for leaving?

Would she give Chrissy the "cold shoulder" as she had done to us in the past when having been away for much shorter periods of time?

Christine expected the worst so her heart wouldn't break if Kailey reacted badly. She knew Kailey was just a 2 year old, but it would still hurt to see that reaction. Christine braced herself as her mom helped her out of our Nissan Xterra. They made their way toward the front door of our house. The door opened.

What happened next was absolutely amazing and will forever be etched in my memory as one of the greatest days of our entire familial life.

Tell me, how do you capture in words, how do you write about your 2 year old daughter, not yet knowing her mom was on the way home, rushing out to the front porch with the biggest smile on her face I have ever seen; not just rushing, but jumping up into the air and clapping.

How do you describe, that from her little mouth came the words, "Yeah, my mommy's home!" and capture the magic of the moment, the vision of what was transpiring.

How do you express with words, the image of my wife being helped to the front porch, barely able to walk under her own power, as her daughter calls out, "Mommy, I missed you so much! I love you so much!" all the while clapping and spinning and jumping as high as her little feet could take her?

How can I even begin to capture the moment of the first hug; the first amazing hug, when Christine struggled to one knee and our daughter smothered her with hugs, resting her little head on mommy's shoulder, left hand lightly patting Christine on her back?

Kailey paid no attention to the mask on Christine's face, or the rubber gloves on her hands. She paid no attention to the tired look in Christine's eyes as the tears ran quickly down her cheeks. All she knew, or cared to know, was that her mommy was home. The moment was precious.

We all just stared at the beauty of what was unfolding before our eyes. How a 2 year old can love her mother unconditionally and with all her heart. How she looked into Christine's eyes after that first amazing hug, and with all the meaning a 2 year old could muster, she asked Christine the question. The question that proved she understood at least a little of what her mom was going through.

She held onto Christine's shoulder with her left hand and bent her head down just a little to look directly into Christine's eyes as she knelt down, and she asked in the cutest little voice," Mom? Your boo boo's all bedda?"

Christine answered, "Yes honey, mommy's boo boo's all better."

Kailey followed with another cheer and we all joined in. I'm sure our neighbors heard the claps and screams of the small party assembled on our front porch.

Tell me though, how do I express in words the look on my daughter's face, right before we went into the house; the look she wore as she yelled, "Everybody's home! I so happy!" and threw her hands up in the air, triumphant?

Later that day, after showing Christine some new things in the house, we all sat in the living room talking. Befitting the warm greeting from our daughter, Kailey ended the afternoon in the perfect way. She climbed up onto the couch next to Christine and buried her nose in Chrissy's ear. Kailey's eyes slowly began to close. She then climbed around to the front of Chrissy, lied down in her lap, and fell asleep in her arms…homecoming miracle complete.

Now tell me, how the hell do you write that, and make it as amazing as the actual moment? You can't.

I could not believe what I saw, and am absolutely convinced that a host of angels guard my wife in every way, each and every day.

Since the homecoming Christine has visited the doctor twice. Both times her blood counts were just about normal and things have been looking good. She is still missing the T-cells though.

Over the last week we decorated the Christmas tree and even put up some decorations around the house. Everything looks great. Christine made decorating easy by buying Christmas storage boxes last year and the year before. I now know where every Christmas decoration is hiding in the attic.

We had to get a fake Christmas tree this year because Chrissy can't have a live one in the house. I hate to admit it, having been a long time live Christmas tree fan, but

I dig not having to hang the lights on the tree and not having the ornaments fall off flimsy braches. I give it an A+ and am fully aware that without the plastic tree we wouldn't have one at all. God bless Christmas tree technology.

Christine has just been overly amazing. She went from needing help walking up and down the stairs when we first got home, to handling the navigation all by herself in just a few days.

Christine now roams the halls daily, doing laps around our dining room, kitchen and foyer. She does get winded quickly and sometimes pushes herself a little too hard, but that comes from being an athlete I think. She is determined to get better faster and pushes herself all the more. I sometimes have to tell her to stop it and sit down. Sometimes she even listens.

Determination: That's my wife. She kept her promise by getting out of the hospital early. She was told 5-8 weeks and she said 3-5. It was exactly 5 weeks on Dec. 8th. She just rocks.

I'm trying to think of anything else I should cover, but I'm just happy to finally have a moment to fill you in on our progress.

Man, I can't tell you how all of your positive energy has helped her through this. The letters, packages, e-mails, calls, prayers, support, everything! It has been amazing.

Christine has begun checking the messages to CareforChristine@yahoo.com herself now. She takes a look on a regular basis and if she's feeling up to it responds back to them.

How do we know she's getting better?

I know Christine is getting better, not just from the blood counts, appetite, and lack of fever. Here's a short bulleted list that I like to call:

The Top 10 Reasons I Know Christine is Getting Better:

10. All of our Christmas gifts are almost wrapped and I didn't do it

9. I have had a "to do" list almost every day in the last week…written out and taped to my forehead.

8. She ate a huge piece of steak yesterday

7. She starts sentences with, "Tom, I'm sorry to be a pain but…" She's not really sorry. I can tell.

6.	We went to see the Christmas lights at the PNC Art Center in NJ and had a blast.

5.	She's called me a 'jerk' at least 7 times in the last 4 days.

4.	She now takes just 6 pills daily and not 106.

3.	Kailey's "fish of anti-nausea" is no longer hanging on our wall.

2.	I've had to say," would you stop cleaning and go sit down!" about 1,000 times

and, the number 1 reason I know Christine is getting better…She snooped around for Christmas gifts and saw one of hers. She lied about it, but couldn't help giving it away with a smile.

Yep, she's getting better alright and with only 7 shopping Days Left until Christmas!

****

The ups and downs continued. We became very used to traveling to the hospital at a moment's notice simply because we could never risk misreading a symptom or being relaxed about something that we didn't perceive as normal. In the following case it was an easy call that she needed to return to the hospital as soon as possible. Thank goodness it was after Christmas. Christmas at home was the best one ever. Santa had brought us more than gifts this year.

<u>Day 46, Monday, December 29, 2003:</u>

Our Christmas was fantastic and we enjoyed every moment of being home together for the holidays. We laughed, cried and loved like a family should.

Christine enjoyed every moment of being in our home even without being able to do anything. Being in a hospital for 5 weeks can make you appreciate a lot of things. Being home, in a place you helped create; a place you made comfortable in your own way; a place where your 2 year old daughter feels safe and sound, creates one of the best feelings in the world.

We decorated the house and had a great Christmas Eve in our home with our immediate family. It was a lot of work, but it was great to have everyone in one place celebrating together.

Kailey loved all her presents and we think her favorite toy was the Fisher Price Doll House we, I mean Santa, brought her this year. She plays with it daily.

We received a number of wonderful Christmas cards this year. A lot of inspirational words and prayers for a happy and healthy 2004 arrived for our family. Thanks so much for your thoughts and continued prayers.

Back in the Hospital

Christine has been back in the hospital since Saturday morning [Dec 27, 2003] at 6AM. She woke up at 5AM and vomited. Her temperature was 101.6 degrees. We called the hospital and got her in right away. They checked her out and admitted her.

It turns out Christine has a bacterial infection in her blood. She has been receiving antibiotics since Saturday and her fever has been under control since Saturday evening.

Christine will remain in the hospital until they can determine exactly what kind of bacteria she has and they can give her the specific antibiotic to fight that type of germ. We're both hoping she can leave very soon, especially in time for New Year's. Keep your fingers crossed and keep praying for her.

We love you and Happy Holidays.

****

When a patient gets repeated IV or the veins in someone's arms are used frequently enough they can often wear out or even collapse, making it difficult to take blood from them or give medicine. This was the case with Christine and because of the number of drugs and blood tests still required the doctors decided to have medical ports surgically implanted in Christine to make the process easier. The ports connected from her chest [Hickman catheter] and arm [Hoan catheter] directly into larger veins in her body. One catheter even connected directly to her heart. These catheters must be diligently cared for to avoid infection at the point of entry or even worse, infection of a main vein or something as critical as the heart. Christine's mom and I took very good care of her catheters. Her mom, twice as much as me, while I was at work. Sometimes, despite all the effort, if they're left in long enough something is bound to happen.

<u>**Day 47, Tuesday, December 30, 2003:**</u>

Christine is being released from the hospital tomorrow after a short 4 and a half day stay. Her fever has not shown itself since late Saturday evening and her current vomiting is due to the anesthesia from having her catheter removed.

The catheter had bacteria in each of its 3 ports and the decision was made to remove the "Hickman" catheter and replace it with a smaller uninfected "Hoan" catheter. [Since the Hickman goes directly into the heart an infection here can be extremely dangerous.]

Christine would normally be able to receive the remaining IV medicine through a normal vein injection, but her veins aren't what they used to be since she had so many problems with her platelets earlier in her treatments and needed so many transfusions. They're all worn out.

The good news is we'll all be able to spend New Year's Eve together and be with our baby to ring in the New Year. Thank goodness!

Christine will be on IV antibiotics at home for the next 12 days or so. We'll learn how to administer the antibiotics through a home nursing service. That will alleviate additional hospital time and frustration for her.

Christine will also begin taking preventative treatments for a form of pneumonia that usually shows itself between days 70 and 80. This will be given through a breathing nebulizer similar to those used for people with asthma.

We are so happy to leave the hospital tomorrow, especially since Kailey has been asking for us daily and nightly. The trip into the hospital at 5AM on Saturday didn't afford us the opportunity to say goodbye to K. She's been missing us a lot, which is nice to hear, but can also break your heart.

In case I can't get another message out before the ball drops, we'd like to wish you a healthy, happy, and blessed 2004. Happy New Year everyone!

****

As mentioned earlier, every small milestone was a big deal. Another major milestones was called "Reaching Day 100."   I write more about Day 100 a little later on but mention it in the following passage.

Day 54, Tuesday, January 6, 2004:

First of all "Happy New Year!" (again). We have been enjoying our time at home since Christine was released from the hospital on New Year's Eve. We were home by about 1PM and enjoyed a nice quiet New Year's Eve with each other.

Kailey made it until about 11:15PM but by then "she had no power captain!" She was out like a light and we put her into bed. Christine and I watched the ball fall in Time Square, sitting on the couch next to one another. We were happy to see the end of 2003, and excited to see the coming of a new year.

We both cried a little and we hugged a lot.

Christine has been home recuperating and her mom and I have been giving her her antibiotics and taking her through her breathing treatments.

We each gained another notch on our medical belt by learning how to administer the IV antibiotic Cipro. Christine is taking Cipro due to her last fever that sent her to the hospital. When you take an antibiotic it's important to finish the whole cycle to ensure you kill the infection. She completes her last dose of Cipro on January 10th, HER 30th BIRTHDAY!!!!

We will spend a nice quiet night home again, but it sure as hell beats time in the hospital. For everyone's information, I am not yet 30. Therefore, I am in fact married to an older woman. I love rubbing it in for at least a few days until my birthday on January 26th.

Christine started taking a preventative treatment called Pentamidine to fight a form of pneumonia, which usually presents itself at around day 70 to 80. By going through these breathing treatments Christine will avoid this sickness. Her mom learned the process from the visiting nurse service and is helping her with those treatments.

Today is day 54, so we are making our way slowly and steadily to Day 100!

Christine, Kailey and I would like to once again wish everyone a Happy and Healthy 2004. God bless you all for your thoughtfulness throughout last year. We have renewed and continued many friendships through your love and support, especially through communications with the website and the Care for Christine Support Network.

We thank you all for a very successful 2003 and look forward to enjoying an even more successful 2004.

****

As Christine took her medicines to get better and to prevent potential complications, a couple of friends began their push to raise money for The Leukemia & Lymphoma Society (LLS) by participating in one of their remarkable programs called Team in Training (TNT). This program supports individuals preparing for events like half or full marathons and triathlons. In return, participants raise money for cancer research and patient services. Without the help and research of organizations like LLS my wife might not have been alive to see her 30th birthday. For that reason, I will continue to support LLS and other causes that combat leukemia and other cancers. Keep running guys and gals. Keep running.

Day 58, Saturday, January 10, 2004:

Happy Birthday Christine!

Today, January 10th, is Christine's 30th birthday. 30 years ago today my little lady was born.

She enjoyed her birthday on our couch, watching TV and waiting patiently for 4:30PM to roll around so she could begin watching football. Or was that me?

As a husband I can tell you it's great to see the circle of friends my wife has around her. I would like to send a personal "Thank You" to everyone who sent birthday cards, food, presents, cakes, e-mails, and phone calls.

Christine is right this very minute taking her last dose of Cipro, the antibiotic she has been taking to fight the infection that put her in the hospital after Christmas.

Cipro made Christine feel sick in the beginning, but we started running the IV drip a little slower. She seemed to tolerate it better that way.

In case the doctor is reading this, don't worry, it always finishes between an hour and an hour and a half.

Day 58 is here as we move our way closer to day 100, our next major milestone. Christine is now taking three different medicines; Gama Globulin (sp?), rituxan, and a breathing medicine called Pentamidine, along with her standard daily set of pills.

As mentioned, the Pentamidine is to fight a type of pneumonia that could develop post-transplant.

The Rituxan is to help fight a potential lymphoma or other Epstein Barr virus complication.

The Gama Globulin is to help boost her immune system until it gets stronger.

Christine will be taking each of these medications for about another 4 months, but they're given with different frequencies. Christine also takes some other pills to help keep her healthy and prevent virus, infections, and bacteria, but these are a lot easier to take than the IV drips and breathing apparatus.

Moving in the Right Direction

Christine continues to move in the right direction and she gets stronger every day. Christine's hair is starting to come back, and although it looks dark, if you look closely you can see a little blonde in there. It may be too early to tell the exact color.

Run Anthony Run! [Another friend running for the cause!]

A good friend and former college teammate of mine, Anthony Bartolomeo, will be running a marathon in Orlando Florida to benefit the Leukemia & Lymphoma Society. Anthony is a former wide receiver and safety for the Georgetown University Football Team.

Anthony raised over $4,000 for LLS in order to participate in the marathon as a member of LLS' Team in Training program. 26.2 miles is a helluva long way to run, and we wish him our best.

It's both an honor and a pleasure to have someone run in Christine's name. When Anthony crosses the finish line tomorrow, he will have "Happy Birthday Christine!" written across the front of his "Team in Training" T-shirt.

On that note, don't forget my pal Steve who will be running a marathon for the same Team in Training program in Arizona. (http://www.stevetornello.com)

Thanks again to all our friends and family. Your support and thoughtfulness continues to help us to get better day by day.

****

An uneventful day is a good thing when you're recovering from a BMT. This update also included one of the many notes that touched our hearts. People were making a big difference in keeping Christine positive during her recovery.

Day 61, Tuesday, January 13, 2004:

Christine is doing well but is beginning to get sick of sitting in the house. If the weather was nicer she'd be able to take some walks and maybe build up a little more energy, but with all this cold weather she must resort to days filled with Noggin [children's TV channel] and the Disney Channel. She keeps in mind that no news is good news and uneventful is synonymous with "out of the hospital" so she will bide her time until she's allowed to party again.

Our friend Anthony finished the Orlando Marathon in 4 hours 32 minutes. God bless people with big hearts and good lungs. Great job!

A Letter from Anthony

Dear Tom,

First of all I want to say happy belated B-day to Christine!!! I did it! I finished all 26.2 miles in 4 hours and 32 minutes. It was by far the hardest athletic feat I have ever accomplished. There were a lot of ups and downs along the way but overall it was an amazing experience or as they would say in Disney, a magical experience…

…I hope all is well and be sure to give Christine my love, I hope she enjoyed her birthday as much as I enjoyed the opportunity to run with her name on my shirt.

Talk to you soon,
Anthony

****

As the Day-100 milestone approached and Christine seemed to be getting better I felt more and more like I was on top of the world.

<u>Day 90, Tuesday, February 11, 2003:</u>

Christine continues to do well and day 100 is quickly approaching.

Day 100 will not bring the luxuries it would if it came during the summer time, but we do get to go out a little more. The Doctor said the winter time is difficult to venture out safely due to all the illnesses that go around. It also has been particularly bad for the flu and other cold-related illnesses this year, so we have to watch ourselves. I think we both think it'll feel kind of funny going out again for the first time in such a long time. Almost like a first date but with a kid in tow. We're looking forward to it!

Christine is still taking one of two medications every other week. Next week she gets Rituxan and last week she received a new drug called IVIG.

Rituxan helps to subdue the Epstein Barr virus until Christine's strong enough to fight it herself, and IVIG helps strengthen her immune system until it progresses further on its own.

I know there's a lot of talk about her blood counts being normal, but Christine doesn't have her full immune system back yet. Her blood counts are all in the normal range; however, her white blood cells are still missing pieces to them. Her last white count was 6.2, which is great, but there are 4-5 different types of white blood cells and not all of them are back yet.

The T-Cells, which are a white "fighter" blood cell, are lower than they need to be so that's what we're waiting on. (Another Example: the B white cells are where the EBV virus dwells, so the Rituxan treatments suppress the B cells to try and prevent the virus from advancing to something like EBV Lymphoma.)

Christine and I are looking forward to this spring and summer when we can get out of the house and do some fun things. She's also looking forward to doing things with other members of our family and friends we haven't seen in a while. She may even be joining the Menoni family scrap-book club. That's my mom's side of the family.

Christine has stayed busy. I've never seen her on the computer as much as I have these last few weeks. The new PC was a great idea as she checks her messages regularly and replies to them when she can.

Christine loves getting updates from you all and those who have continually kept in touch with regular messages "thanks!" and keep'em coming.

Our daughter Kailey can just about count to 20 if you count it "13, 14, 16, 15, 19, 20." She is such a doll I can't take it. We've been playing with her an awful lot and Chris and I are happy she's been able to play outside a few times in the last week or so.

A Doctor's work is never done

We'd like to take an opportunity to thank someone who spends their life dedicated to saving lives. Dr. Ann Jakubowski of MSKCC has been Christine's primary leukemia and transplant doctor throughout her 2 years of treatment. A lot more than just offering care goes into her role, including answering countless questions, giving advice, telling it like it is, knowing the facts, knowing her patients, caring a lot about those she's curing and being there when you need someone at that level to look up to when the going gets tough.

We heard great things about Dr. J before we started treatments back in March 2002 and we can say for a fact that she has been an amazing doctor and more importantly, a remarkable person.

Dr. Ann Jakubowski, I thank you, Christine thanks you, Kailey thanks you, our families thank you, and the Care for Christine Support Network thanks you for everything you've done so far and will continue to do. The world needs more people like you!

Christine's Experience Helps Others

It makes me happy and proud when our family makes a positive impact on someone's life. The website was originally meant to update friends and family on Christine's progress and I can truly say it's been that and so much more. We have built a support network of well over 200 families strong.

I was recently told by someone in the network that someone who was recently diagnosed with leukemia and is going through treatments has been using Christine's website to get information on the disease and to help put things in perspective. I'm told that using Christine's experiences for guidance has helped. We pray that anyone who can use the site for strength and purpose do so with our full blessing.

Each day this ever changing world brings an uncertainty that we'd never felt before Christine's illness, but it also brings a sense of happiness we had never known.

This experience has taken 'life' and made it........LIFE! (and we're just getting started all over again:-)

****

It was interesting to see how many little things all of a sudden meant so much. Every little experience became time we got to spend together as a family. Something as simple as running an errand was "family time." At times though, we felt like outlaws on the run as we ran from place to place, Christine always waiting patiently for me in the car with a mask and gloves on. I don't think she ever got used to the stares from people in other cars as we drove. I remember one time she asked, "Why does everyone have to stare?" and I answered. "It's not every day you get to see a beautiful woman in a mask and gloves driving in the car next to you." That got me a smile every time. We tried to keep it as light as we could.

Day 93, Friday, February 14, 2003:

(Valentine's Day)

From Christine, Kailey and I, Happy Valentine's Day Everyone!

Christine continues to do well and it looks like she'll have her catheter removed in the next week or so. That will significantly reduce a potential site of infection.

The Hoan Catheter that Christine has been receiving her meds through can be taken out without surgery right in the doctor's office, so it will be cool to get it out once and for all.

They can remove the catheter because the nurses in the adult day hospital say her veins are good enough again to give her IV medication. They had been worried that Christine's veins had gone through too much with all the blood transfusions, but they liked what they saw when they examined her. Plus, there are only 2 medications she's now receiving through IV, and they're monthly.

So we're on day-93 and it couldn't be any better. Christine is moving along nicely and today has been fantastic. We opened Valentine's Day gifts, ate pancakes for breakfast, sang, danced a little, cried a little and enjoyed our time together. I skipped a Saturday morning class [work related] to spend the full day with Chrissy and Kailey.

We have some running around to do today, but it's funny how the running around has become our weekly outing and we look forward to getting out of the house as a family.

Jenn's Wedding!

We'd like to wish our cousin Jennifer good luck and congratulations on her wedding day! You'll probably see Christine poking her head out the car window as you get out of the limo! But of course, you're not reading this right now because you're prepping for the wedding.

OK, this was a quick Valentine's Day update. God bless and keep smiling.

****

The following update is from one of the proudest days of my life. It's right up there with my wedding day and the day our daughter was born. This was such a fantastic milestone to reach and what happened on Feb 21 befit a fairy tale. I'll let the update speak for itself.

Day 100!!!, Friday, February 21, 2003:

Congratulations Christine on hitting DAY 100!!! We're all so proud of you!!! YES! Today, Saturday Feb 21st is Day 100!!!

You heard it correctly! In case you didn't have your calendar marked, today is the 100th day since Christine's BMT and a MAJOR milestone on her road to recovery!

We are all so proud of her that we had a hard time containing ourselves. To fully appreciate the day you really need to have the picture in your head of Christine with a smile on from ear to ear.

There was something magical, something amazing in the air; an electricity that could be felt as we both opened our eyes this morning in bed. Although it may have been generated by the white of Christine's smile, I think it was a combination of many things. The recipe may have went something like this:

10 parts love, 10 parts prayer, 5 parts hope, 1000 parts family, 20.5 parts joy, and a pinch of a whole mess of other things along the same line.

When I opened my eyes this morning the first thing I saw was Kailey lying next to us in bed and just beyond her was my wife with that smile, staring at me like it was Christmas morning. It woke me up more than a first cup of coffee.

From the time we opened our eyes it was only minutes before the three of us were in the back bedroom ready to celebrate. It was 8:30AM and the sun found the cracks in the blinds lighting the room like the heavens through the clouds. We almost didn't know what to do with ourselves. The emotions ran through us.

Christine went to the computer and put on the first song.

We danced. The three of us, moving around the room with our best 8:30AM dance moves. We smiled at each other, almost laughed defiantly, as Gloria Gaynor sang "I Will Survive," Christine's choice, in memory of a dear friend watching down over us.

The next song that filled the room was one I had played for Chrissy many times in the last three months. The Beatles sang "Here Comes the Sun" for us. We danced this one close together; Kailey in my arms and Christine in Kailey's arms; swaying back and forth as the words rang true to our ears.

"Little darling, it's been a long cold lonely winter; little darling it feels like years since it's been here. Here comes the sun...."

We danced and danced and I caught Christine's eye as Kailey put her head on Christine's shoulder. The tears were coming and I couldn't help but choke up as it sounded once again as if Paul McCartney was singing to us personally; singing as if the words were meant for us, right at that moment on Day-100.

"Little darling, the smiles returning to the faces. Little darling, it feels like years since it's been here. Here comes the sun..."

We hugged as we swayed for much of the 3 minutes it took for Paul to sing us the story of the sun coming back into our lives and the light that we were walking toward with each and every minute that passed.

"Little darling, I feel the ice is slowly melting. Little darling, it feels like years since it's been clear. Here comes the sun. Here comes the sun. I say, it's alright..."

And the words faded into my mind like a message from a distant place. Christine and I said a lot to each other during that song, a lot without speaking. Our tear filled eyes did all the talking. Kailey knew the moment was special. When the song ended she continued to hug Christine with her head still on Chrissy's shoulder.

"I love you mom." was all she said.

The third song we danced to has been Chrissy's staple song ever since I heard it walking to the hospital well over a year ago.

It was during her first round of treatments in 2002 and I knew once I heard it that my Chrissy was going to be alright. Jimmy Eat World sings an amazing song called "The Middle."

"It just takes some time little girl, you're in the middle of the ride. Everything will be just fine, everything, everything will be alright."

It's an upbeat song that makes you want to jump through the ceiling with confidence. Christine had to relax herself as she boogied it up with Kailey and me. She reminded herself she was still recovering and wasn't ready for a dance marathon, so we went downstairs together.

It wasn't even 9AM and the day had been incredible. I will remember those dances, that half hour of complete and utter joy, all the days of my life.

I've said it many times already, but I can't help but restate how amazing life has become for us. We have learned so much through this experience and feel happy to have another chance at making our dreams come true. Those dreams have changed a great deal over the last three years and happiness and success have been redefined a number of ways. Before Christine became sick I can't say we weren't focused on the material things in life just a little too much; sometimes maybe even more than a little. We now look at our family and the time we spend together as our true gauge of success.   By putting our family at the center of our lives we feel the rest of the chips begin to fall into place. It's not always perfect by any means. We still have the same family struggles as most, but having our family at the center, and understanding how valuable this time together is, helps us to get through it all. Even more important is actually realizing how quickly all of this can be taken away without warning. Our dreams, happiness and success keep being redefined as we see Christine continue her recovery, as we see our daughter grow, as we see our individual friends and family begin their own families and as we deal with the hardships that life brings us each and every day. I think when this is over I will write a book. I will call it...To There and Back Again...A Family's Journey.

I already think I have the perfect ending for our story...' and [we] lived happily ever after.'

Day 100 Dinner Celebration

Christine and our family went out for an early dinner today to celebrate Day 100. One new activity Christine can partake in is eating out at a nice clean restaurant during an off-peak hour. She chose one of her favorite Italian Restaurants close to our house [on Staten Island]. The food was great. Christine was so excited! It was an awesome feeling.

When I got home from running errands earlier in the day, Christine was nervously getting ready. It was like we were going on a first date, except we're married, have a child and both our families were with us. She was sooooo cute as she got ready. She kept telling me how she couldn't believe how nervous she was.

We began dinner at about 3PM and although Christine couldn't eat the shrimp parmesan she's been craving (due to a shrimp restriction), she went with eggplant parm and spaghetti, another of her favorites.

Kailey was absolutely thrilled to have everyone out with her and she kept milling about like she was the hostess. As we left the restaurant she screamed to all the patrons, "Bye everybody!" and waved. What a ham.

We would like to thank the restaurant for opening their dining room up an hour earlier for us. The extra hour allowed us to eat before the crowd came in. It was very nice of them to do that for us.

After dinner Christine, Kailey and I went back to Christine's parents' house to have birthday cake for her grandmother, Nana who turned 87 years young today.

Here's a quick update on Christine's week at the hospital:

We arrived at the hospital early on Wednesday because school was out and it didn't snow as predicted, but that ensured an early start. Christine was seen by her doctor and her blood counts looked fantastic. Everything was in the normal ranges. We reviewed some of the extra things she can now do since reaching day 100. The most significant of the new activities is going out to eat with small groups of people as long as no one is sick, exposed to someone who's sick, or think they may be getting sick.

Christine then went for a bone marrow biopsy, which is when a needle is inserted into the hip bone located at around the lower back. Christine hates this test the most and usually has trouble sleeping 2-3 nights before because of anxiety. This was the case this time as well.

The main purpose of the bone marrow biopsy is to collect "baby" blood cells to confirm that the donor's blood is growing in Christine and to see if any of her own blood is still growing as well. It is also to confirm that her blood is clean. This test usually takes 3-4 weeks for results to return because they are done at the DNA or chromosome level after an initial "naked eye" analysis is done by the doctor under the microscope.

After the biopsy Christine had her monthly treatment of Rituxan that she will get for another three months or so.

Before the Rituxan, the nurse checked Christine's veins to make sure they looked good enough to give blood and receive medication. She gave blood through a vein in her hand and received the Rituxan through the same without any issues.

Because of this, Chrissy had the central line removed from her chest.

The Hoan Catheter is out! This is now one less source of possible infection! Woooo Whoooo!!!

To finish off the long day Christine met with one or two other doctors for various things and then she went home, exhausted, but relieved it was over. The next day she was like a new person. It was great to see.

We will continue to go to the doctor every two weeks for her standard check-ups. She will have some additional tests coming up here and there, but I will be sure to report back on any of the major ones.

Angels for Christine Unite!!!

It's that time of year again folks. We are beginning to prepare for this year's Light The Night walk to raise money for the Leukemia & Lymphoma Society. This will be the THIRD year in a row that the Angels for Christine will be entering a team to do the walk.

Day 100 Conclusion!

What a day! Christine was so excited for me to write about the 100th day and let everyone know how she's doing.

I am so proud of her and her accomplishments, words are impossible to express it. She keeps on smiling and keeps on getting better. Our next major milestone is the six month mark. I know it seems like a long way off, but so was Day 100 when we first started.

In closing, I'd just like to thank you all again. As a caring husband, I can tell you that your support helps keep up my strength in giving Christine the support she needs. I can honestly say that this has made us a stronger family. It has strengthened friendships and opened our eyes to a whole new world, an amazing new world that we've been staring at for years and just never realized.

In the words of other people:

"Little darling, the smiles returning to the faces."

"Everything will be just fine. Everything will be alright."

"And they lived happily ever after."

Hey everyone,"Here comes the sun"

****

As Christine continued to get better there was more to learn and it kept us on our toes. We tried to be as close to perfect as possible, following every rule and guideline the doctors and nurses gave us to the tee. We paid attention to every detail. It was what we needed to do to keep sharp. When we learned more I tried to relay the information. I took a look back at all the obstacles we had overcome since late 2001. Looking back I guess we felt like dominos waiting for the next bad break to fall and knock us down. Writing about our experiences brought the world into perspective. We'll never forget what we went through to be together today. We also wanted people to see that if we could do it, anyone could do it.

Day 117, Sunday, March 9, 2003:

Well, today is Day 117 and things have been going nicely since our grand old day-100 celebration. Christine has been getting stronger and feeling better each day. There are some occasions where she'll feel very tired during the day and early evening, but that's still to be expected. Most of the time Christine can now make it until 9PM without feeling extremely tired; by 10PM though she's ready for bed. That seems pretty standard. 10PM is a lot later than 2PM, when she used to hit the proverbial brick-wall shortly after coming home from the hospital.

Since our day-100 dinner we've ordered food to the house quite a few times. Chrissy's eating habits have gotten a lot better and she is maintaining her weight, which is very important at this stage of the game. Her favorite food right now seems to be a tie between the spinach and broccoli rolls.

We also had a really nice meal at a steakhouse in Great Kills down by the water last weekend. We stopped there after a walk on the beach and a stroll through the park. It was 3PM and only one other table was occupied in the restaurant. While we were eating, 3 other parties came in and Christine started to get a little nervous. Dining out again is going to take a little getting used to, but hopefully practice will make perfect.

Strolls on the beach and in the park have been some of our favorite thing to do. Yes, Staten Island still has beaches that you can walk on. As a matter of fact they're a lot nicer than they were 10 years ago.

It's amazing how calm the soft rush of the ocean can make you feel and simultaneously how nerve wracking it can be watching Kailey by the edge of the water. I think the words, "Kailey back up!" will forever be etched in my memory.

We went for a walk there last weekend as well as today. It was also nice to watch Kailey play in the little playground at the park by the beach. Christine and I were so happy to see her having a good time. One of the best moments had to be right before it was her turn to go down the slide. She would look down at us and ask, "Can I go now?" We'd give her the thumbs up and she'd say with a big excited smile, "MOM, DAD! Watch me go down the slide!" The little things...

Visitors

We've had some visitors over the last two weeks. Friends and family, who hadn't been able to come by prior to Day 100, called and arranged short visits to say hello. Unfortunately, we haven't been able to say yes to everyone and we're being very strict about the illness thing. We can't take any chances. Thanks to everyone who's been patient with our strict visitation policy, but this is very very important.

Doctor Visits

Christine has had a couple of doctor visits since the last message but this coming week is a big one. On Wednesday Christine goes in for a lumbar puncture. That's a nice way of saying spinal tap. She will need one spinal tap a month for roughly six months. The reason for this procedure is this: leukemia, and more specifically Christine's leukemia, which presented itself outside of her bone marrow and in her circulating blood, can possibly find its way into the spinal fluid and hide out there. The spinal fluid and nervous system, in general, have a unique build which separates and segregates them from the bulk of infections and diseases that attack the body on an everyday basis. The segregation also happens with chemotherapy. Unfortunately, blood cancers, like leukemia, have a chance of making it into the nervous system because they look a lot like normal cells. They can sometimes fake their way into the nervous system and hide away. To fight the chances of relapse due to leukemia in the spinal fluid these spinal taps are necessary. The purpose is twofold:

1) To take a sample of the spinal fluid to make sure there are no leukemia cells present.

2) To introduce chemotherapy into the spinal fluid to kill any lingering leukemia

cells should they be present and not detected.

The good news is the last time Christine had this test done, roughly a year ago, there was no leukemia present. The not-so-good news is after the last spinal tap Christine had very bad headaches and threw up for a day and a half. Of course, Christine is very nervous about this test, one she hates even more than the bone marrow biopsies. We're hoping that because Christine's platelet counts are normal this time around she'll be just fine. Say a couple of extra prayers for her this week.

Next Milestone:

The next milestone for Christine is the 6 month mark. As we're already on Day 117 we're only 2 months and 5 days away. This is so exciting and with raw determination we look forward to hitting each new milestone. My new favorite thing to do at the doctor's office is to ask Dr. Jakubowski if Christine can do certain things. I love it because every once in a while I will throw in something absolutely outrageous and the doctor will look at me in disbelief. I also say things like, "I think Christine overdid it the other day when she was washing the cars..." The doctor will sometimes look at Christine like she wants to kill her a split second before I say, "Just kidding." The doctor will probably get tired of this new game really soon, but knowing myself I "just won't know when to stop," which I've heard since the first grade. We did get a good laugh when Christine asked the doctor if she can eat sushi. The doctor laughed at that one too and said, "Aaaaaaah....no." It was pretty funny. It was encouraging to hear that she'll be able to feast on lobster and shrimp in the near future though. Shellfish is still in the "red zone," but will soon be on the acceptable foods menu.

****

As I read through the updates I realize beyond any shadow of a doubt, that writing was my outlet. It was my therapy while it seemed everything was crumbling down around us. It wasn't just Christine's illness, it was so much more than that. It was the seemingly non-stop onslaught of tragedy that hit our family and friends beginning in 2001. Sometimes, the only way to plan a strategy or even a simple way forward is to reflect, and take inventory of what's happening around you. To defeat an enemy, you first need to look him in the eyes.

My Reflection…

My family has been through a lot in the last few years. If anyone told me that by the age of 30 I'd have witnessed my loved ones go through such tough times I would have never believed it. If anyone told me I'd travel these rough roads alongside the ones I love I'd have thought them insane.

It started back in 2001. The happiest moment of my life, the birth of my daughter on August 3rd, was followed by one of the most horrific acts of terrorism just over a month later. I lost one of my best friends that day as well as a number of other people I grew up with. I miss my buddy Joey dearly and not a day goes by that I don't speak to him. I know he's listening. Christine lost her close friend Sharon in a car accident a few months later, on Christmas morning. Christine prays to her often and finds solace in the signs Sharon sends her from up above. Joey and Sharon were our age and they were both part of our wedding party. Taken too early; our hearts wept and still do to this day.

2002 was supposed to be a happier time. A better year, but Christine was diagnosed in March and our personal battle began. Since then it's been an up and down struggle. We have our good times and bad times and help each other up when we're down. We have amazing support from friends and family and that has helped keep the momentum going our way. There are no other options so our thankfulness is overwhelming. We will continue to fight and we will win this war against leukemia one battle at a time.

As I think about the cruelties that life can bring to each and every family when they seem to least expect it, I feel the same anger that built inside when I found that Christine had relapsed this past summer; the same "HOW CAN YOU DO THIS TO US!" anger that made me begin to question my faith. That kind of thinking needs to be short lived though, when faith and hope are all you have left. Instead, I took that anger and turned it into strength; the strength I needed to do whatever I could to be there for Christine as she went through the hardest parts of her treatment; the strength to smile when I wanted to cry; the strength to wake up in the morning and do what I needed to do to make us a little better than we were the day before. I use that same strength to write every update on my wife's progress, even when she got sicker before my eyes. Instead of shouts of doubt we turned it into "defiant progress" as we moved forward. We're still going strong. Be sure that we had help along the way; my parents, Christine's parents, our close friends and family, and all of you reading this update on Chrissy's progress. You all are a part of the strength that keeps us moving.

Many a road has been traveled on angels' wings. They're all around us and waiting to help us out. Don't forget to ask. Stay strong, stay tough, chins up, and God bless.

****

There was never a dull moment when a spinal tap was involved. It didn't seem to matter what they did to ease the side effects. Christine and spinal taps just didn't mix.

<u>Day 121, Saturday, March 13, 2004:</u>

Christine went in for her spinal tap on Wednesday, also known as a "lumbar puncture." We were in early to take a blood test (8AM) and her counts looked great. So at about 9:45AM she went in for the procedure and at 10:15AM she was out of the room. They did the procedure in radiology because the last time she had one of these tests she had massive headaches for 3 days and threw up for a day and a half. Radiology has a more precise method of performing the spinal tap. They take pictures of her insides through a cat scan or some type of x-ray and they actually make sure they stick the needle into the right spot to draw the spinal fluid. My little sweetie said it didn't hurt as much as the bone marrow biopsies she gets every couple of months. The only discomfort was when they gave her the numbing medicine (lidocaine) and when the needle hit a nerve and sent a tiny electric shock down her leg. The shock lasted a very short time though and before she knew it the spinal tap was complete. They put a needle into her spinal region in her lower back and drew fluid to test for leukemia, and they also injected her spinal fluid with chemotherapy to kill anything that might be hiding out, even if leukemia doesn't show up. She'll need those spinal taps once every month for roughly 5 more months.

After the procedure Christine was doing all right. The procedure called for her to lay flat for 2 hours after it was complete. So she laid flat from 10:15AM until 12:45PM and was then released. We left the hospital at about 1:00PM and went home to rest.

Christine was doing fabulous. She ate Denino's pizza (2 slices of the best pizza in the world) and a couple of Buffalo wings at 2PM. She relaxed on the couch and slept for a couple of hours. Then it happened at about 4PM. She vomited and began to get a headache. Christine puked every 15 minutes for the next 2.5 hours. We had to rush back to the hospital and we went right into the emergency room. This was about 6:30PM and by now her headache was so severe she couldn't open her eyes. Christine had lost a lot of fluid and she needed to be re-hydrated through IV since she couldn't hold anything down. We were in the urgent care dept until about 11PM. Then we went home and as exhausted as can be, we slept.

Christine's mom and dad had watched Kailey when we rushed out to the hospital and she was sleeping by the time we got home. When I woke up for work in the morning Kailey was in bed lying between the two of us. It was a nice feeling.

****

Sometimes the updates were more about how other people have touched our lives. Reflection helped us identify the things we had taken for granted for so long. I felt as if my eyes were finally open.

Day 122, Wednesday, March 14, 2004:

Christine felt a lot better than she did on Wednesday night but she still had a little headache and didn't feel herself for most of the day. The frustrating part about procedures like [spinal taps] is you go in feeling fine and you come out feeling like gum on the bottom of a shoe. You're not feeling badly because you're sick. You're feeling badly because of something you did voluntarily. It's so frustrating. But the unfortunate thing is that seems to be the philosophy behind cancer treatments; you hurt yourself to heal yourself. "Cancer treatment", add that to your list of oxymorons right next to "jumbo shrimp" and "dark light." (Christine would now tell me to stop being a geek.)

Cute Story Involving Puke:

There is a cute and somewhat touching story that came out of Christine's puking escapade yesterday. It's funny because it's great seeing how kids react to seeing something for the first time. When Christine began throwing up on Wednesday, Kailey Anne was with us in the living room. Christine had her head buried in a bucket and I was sitting next to her rubbing her back and watching Kailey. She was beginning to get visibly upset that her mommy seemed to be in pain. She stood there moving her feet as if she wanted to go somewhere but didn't know where to go. She asked, "Mommy, are you alright?" and when Christine couldn't immediately answer she looked at me and said, "Daddy, what's wrong with Mommy?" I began to comfort her and Christine did too, as much as possible. Kailey did not have a great angle of Christine's face however and didn't really see what was going on but our comforting words seemed to work and Kailey started nervously smiling a little as I explained. Then it was over and Kailey started to play with her doll-house.

15 minutes later, when Christine began to vomit again, Kailey ran over to help. This time she got closer to Christine's front and saw her vomit into the bucket. Kailey looked at me and walked toward me with a stunned look on her face and involuntarily gagged. It was the funniest and cutest thing to happen at such a weird time. This probably doesn't make sense to a lot of you, but to see the face of a 2.5 year old look up at you so innocently...it warmed my heart. The look was one of, "what did I just see?" Even funnier was when I told Christine about it today she laughed hard. At the worst times you sometimes have to find the humor in the situation although it's often very difficult.

****

As Christine continued to get better my updates sometimes spread themselves out a little more than I would have liked. The funny thing is we were having so much fun being together that time seemed to fly. I felt myself reflecting more and more on our life and our love. We also kept doing things for the first time all over again.

Day 146, Wednesday, April 7, 2004:

Today is April 7, 2004, but more importantly Day 146. Christine is taking a little more of her life back every day. For the last few weeks she has tried different things, gone different places and taken more baby-steps toward her final goal; to be cured from leukemia. It's a goal we all share together.

A lot has happened since I last wrote. The best news is Christine has been out of the hospital except for scheduled visits and in last week's doctor visit we found that her spinal tap tests came back negative, which is fantastic news. We also found that the last bone marrow biopsy results weren't back yet so we're still waiting for them. The bone marrow biopsy will tell us how much of her current blood is from her old bone marrow and what percent is from the new.

More good news is that she has this whole week off from hospital visits. That's always a blessing and she did a little cheer when she looked at the calendar last weekend and saw nothing on it that said "MSKCC."

As I mentioned earlier, Christine has been doing different things and has gotten additional approvals that she's been waiting for. I have noticed that Christine's doctor does in fact read these updates so to avoid incriminating ourselves I must state that Christine has not done anything she wasn't supposed to do. Dr. Jakubowski can be such a stickler sometimes…but that's why we love her.

Get Your Shrimp Here!

Christine has gotten approval to have shrimp one time. Only once, but she's going to love it. The only problem we see with being able to have a food you've craved for so long is, "how should you have it prepared if you can only have it once?" Christine has yet to indulge and can't decide whether to have the delicious shrimp parmesan at the Italian restaurant or whether to have it cooked at home.

If we have it at home we have to worry about me overcooking it and ruining her only opportunity, at least for the short term. I mean, that's a lot of pressure on a husband. I would have to say, "Sorry the shrimp tastes like rubber honey, and sorry for ruining your only opportunity to eat the only food you've craved for six straight months." In light of the pressure she's still deciding on what she feels most comfortable with.

Right on Target! (Shopping anyone?)

Alright, this is a big one! Christine went shopping last week, in a store for the first time since November 3, 2003! She went with her mom to Target in NJ. The doctor said she could go to stores that weren't crowded at non-peak times. So when I picked up my ringing phone at work at 8:13AM on April 1 and said, "OH MY GOD WHAT'S WRONG!" (because I never got calls that early from home) I was greeted with a cheery and excited voice singing, "I'm going shopping! I'm going shopping!" Christine felt very comfortable and enjoyed every second of the experience.

Grocery Stores are NOT Target-like

We took the extended freedom to another level by visiting the grocery store on Sunday night. We usually do grocery shopping at night and it's not crowded at all, but we quickly noticed that grocery stores are sometimes not very clean. On this particular night, it was just our luck that we were followed down aisles 4 and 5 by a lady who was coughing like she's smoked 3 packs a day for the last 40 years and had a frog in her throat. At one point she practically hopped on Christine's back as we were walking down the aisle since she was walking so close. She even blocked our path while deciding which peanut butter to put in her cart. Funnier than that was when Christine had enough and actually pushed me out of the way and ran down the aisle as the coughing woman approached her in aisle 5.

We eventually skipped a few aisles to put some distance between us and the "germ factory" but the damage was already done. I don't think Christine will be visiting a grocery store for a while, at least until she gets some more time under her belt.

FOOOOD!

Christine is now eating very well and although her portions are still smaller than they used to be, she's eating more frequently. Two months ago Christine would suffer horrible stomach pains from dairy but now she's tolerating dairy products better, although she's far from 100%.

All in all, her activity level has increased and we have gone for walks in the park, around the neighborhood, gone to friends' houses, planned mini-outings and are having a very nice time together as a family. We're still looking at our vacation schedule for this year, but waiting to see what our six-month milestone will bring us. With that being said, next Tuesday is the FIVE-MONTH mark!!! How great is that!? FIVE months already, and although we have a long way to go, it's very encouraging to see how far we've come. It's great to be able to head over to the track at the College of Staten Island (CSI) and watch Kailey run around, her little legs taking 7 steps for every one of mine. It's fun to watch her lose speed as her laughter increases and then accelerate when her laughing fit is coming to a close. It's even more amazing to see my wife walking with us smiling all the way.

Note from the Author:

I was asked an interesting question the other day after making this statement:

"I love Christine."

I was then asked, "How do you know?"

My answer started back 15+ years to when I saw Christine Marie Dragula at a high school dance. I didn't know her name, but I would never forget her face and that shy smile. My explanation continued through years of working together, loving together, competing together, standing side by side together, supporting each other, comforting each other, relying on each other and depending on one another.

My answer ended with where we stand today and the trials we have faced and will continue to face in the coming years, together.

There's a lot that effortlessly went into my answer to that question. What made the moment even nicer was the response.

"Wow."

****

As we got closer to our second major post-transplant milestone of six months I spent time not just reflecting and giving updates, but giving examples of how we were taking bits and pieces of our life back. The emotional and mental healing were proving to take even longer than the physical healing.

Day 152, Tuesday, April 13, 2004:

Today was a great day for Day-152! Today is exactly 5 months since Christine's transplant. It's been 5 months since I was sitting in the hospital room with Christine, broadcasting her BMT home to our family via webcam. It's been just over 5 months since a new life was pushed into my wife's body through a central line into her bloodstream. 5 months since she received the blood of an angel who just so happened to match her blood's chromosomal make-up with a 10 for 10 match on the critical chromosomes; an angel who donated a piece of his own life to save Christine's.

It's pretty powerful stuff. At today's doctor's appointments we found that the blood in Christine's bone marrow showed up as being 100% of the donor's. There had been a chance that some of her blood might still be around.

What this means is that her body is growing 100% of the donor's blood and there are no signs of the leukemic cells!

Christine received her 5th dose of Rituxan and I think that means only one more dose in the protocol. She also has only 2 more doses of IVIG left in the protocol as well. That means she'll be finishing these last 2 big medications in the next month and a half. We're so excited about it!

We will be planning a trip to the Northeast (R.I./Maine) for sometime in the second half of May. Christine received approval from her doctor for one Lobster dinner after she reaches the next milestone of six-months. That will be on May 13th and we can't wait.

Our first trip of the year will be for pure relaxation someplace other than our home. Our house is nice, but having been stuck in it for the greater part of the last 4 months Christine needs some time away.

We hope everyone had a happy and healthy Easter holiday. Easter is always a great time for visiting family and friends and for many, including myself, it's a time of new beginnings. Easter will always have a symbolic meaning of our new beginning and our new chance on life together as a family. Christine, Kailey and I have a second chance at a life together that was almost taken away.

At times it felt like we'd never get to the 5 month mark. At times it felt like the days in the hospital away from Kailey, saying good night via the internet and a web cam would never end. Now I look forward to coming home from work to my wife and daughter. As I walk through the door Kailey is usually waiting under a blanket on the couch hiding from me. She screams a happy scream when I lift her up into my arms and ask for my kiss and hug hello. It's not long before Kailey lies on her stomach and asks me to swing her around. I grab her pants and shirt and give her a whirl. She loves the tickle in her stomach and even Christine smiles a nervous smile as she realizes how much fun we're having despite her daughter flying through the air. It's amazing.

Christine had her shrimp dinner on Good Friday. She chose shrimp cocktail at my aunt's house, which was a fantastic choice, I think my aunt and uncle triple and quadruple washed the shrimp cocktail. Christine was in shrimp heaven, we knew the meal was clean enough for her to eat and I was off the hook with trying to prepare the only thing Christine has craved (besides sushi) since Day 1.

I'm sure as insignificant as shrimp are in the grand scheme of life, she'll always remember that moment. Another small piece of her life taken back.

Christine also got the thumbs up to eat Chinese food at today's doctor appointment. So we had it for dinner tonight, minus the fried rice, which apparently has some kind of bacteria which isn't good for her to eat. She feasted on sesame chicken.

We have a nice weekend planned with some additional outings lined up. Remember, life's too short to fight and hold grudges, so if you're holding one, it's time to let it go. A colleague once told me, "It all depends what means most to you; being right, or your relationship with that person."

Think about it.

****

I can't express how important writing became to not only me, but my wife. I love to write and sometimes did so to keep myself moving forward. Christine loved to read what I had to say and so did others in our support network.

Day 169-170, Friday-Saturday, April 30-May 1, 2004:

I am so grateful that I found writing as a way to help me support Christine through her fight against leukemia. I wish I could bottle what it is that makes me want to write; the things that trigger my emotions and inspire me to put my feelings into words. It's not like a faucet that you can turn on and off, but it definitely is something special.

I think this week brought a number of events and inspirational moments that brought me into the right frame of mind to put "pen to paper." Maybe it's knowing that Christine has only one more Rituxan and one more IVIG treatment before this stage of her recovery is complete and we move onto the next. Maybe it's knowing that the six-month mark is quickly approaching; May 13th is right around the corner.

Maybe I'm excited about our upcoming vacation, or getting to see old friends for the first time in a long time, or seeing Christine's smile, something I felt like I'd never see again.

Maybe it's the songs I hear on the radio or the conversations I hold with friends or colleagues. Maybe it's a thought, or a memory, or a dream, or even a conflict. Maybe it's a little bit of each of those things that drive the inspiration.

Or maybe it's the fact that it's been 169 days since Christine's transplant and I'm sitting in front of my computer knowing my wife and daughter are safe and sound, asleep just a few feet away; knowing I can peek in on each of them, not from behind a mask or through a web cam, but for real. I can walk in and brush a hand across their cheeks, not through a latex glove, or on a picture, or in my dreams. Yep, that's definitely enough to get me in the mood to write.

Christine is doing very well, although, she seems to still be struggling a little with feeling comfortable out of the house. She's getting out, but I can still see she's uncomfortable at times. That means we still take it one step at a time; baby steps, but we keep moving forward, slowly.

Since I last wrote, Christine has made more progress and I am extremely proud of how much strength she has gotten back and how much stamina she has regained. She's a real trooper.

As I mentioned earlier, Christine should be in her last month of the larger treatments. Rituxan and IVIG (considered chemotherapy) have been helping her prevent certain infections and diseases she is at risk for during the first 6 months of her recovery.

May 13th will be exactly 6 months post-transplant. She has her last Rituxan in 2 weeks and her last IVIG in roughly a month. She is still on some other medications until her immune system comes back 100%. That should be sometime between months 12 and 14; sometimes a little earlier, sometimes a little later. I don't really care how long it takes, as long as she gets there.

The most difficult part of our fight at this point is facing the life changing effects something like leukemia can have on your family.

I now know that it doesn't matter how strong you are as a person, watching someone you truly love go through the aftermath of the rigorous treatments of something like a BMT will eventually get to you. It then becomes a matter of how you deal with it when it breaks you down. I'm not talking about one knock down either. I'm talking about the continuous roller-coaster of emotions that have you up one minute and down the next. I'm talking about reaching a milestone one day and then having to watch your wife go through the stressful process of test after test to make sure things are moving along in the right direction.

Then there's the waiting; and the look on your wife's face as you sometimes catch her staring off into nothingness; and I wonder what she's thinking at those moments (although I can probably guess). Then there's the good news that puts us back on the top of the world and the smile that she radiates fills the room with a light never before seen.

Then there's the news that tells her she has a few more days before a needle needs to be drilled into her hip bone to test her bone marrow, or a needle needs to be inserted into her spinal cord to draw fluid, and we're smacked right back into reality; we're still in this fight. I can't tell you how hard it is to see her worry. I wish I could take the worry away sometimes, but something tells me that's something that only time will heal.

I look at the clock and realize we're now on day 170. 170 days since that first push of new bone marrow. My God.

At moments like this I'm always glad I keep the words of the late and great Vince Lombardi on hand and we keep "getting up." Vince also said,"The greatest accomplishment is not in never falling, but in rising again after you fall." We plan on it.

****

It was shortly before I wrote the following update that Christine's cousin Jessica wrote an extremely thoughtful and touching essay as part of a college project. Her words were beautiful. It's an honor to be able to include it as part of our story.

Day 179, Monday, May 10, 2004, Mother's Day:

Happy Mother's Day to all you moms out there! We had a great day of planting our annual Mother's Day flowers. We were able to get out and visit with moms who live locally and were able to speak to the moms who lived further away. So, all were accounted for on this beautiful day, where the weather held out and the sun shined for 95% of the morning and afternoon. The Mets avoided a sweep by the Brewers, the Yankees came back to beat the Mariners, and at 10PM after I told Kailey she had to start eating more at breakfast, lunch and dinner because she wanted something the eat, she told me, "What are you talking about dad, my stomach's growling!" I couldn't stop laughing.

We have a Wednesday doctor appointment and Christine gets her last dose of Rituxan (YIPEE!)then Thursday is the six-month mark! We can't wait to once again ask the doctor if Christine can eat sushi even though we know the answer will be "no." Raw fish is pretty risky. We have about 100 other questions that are more practical so we are looking forward to Wed.   Christine has gotten some great messages from friends she hasn't seen in a while; e-mail and technology have proven once again to be an amazing catalyst in helping to bring people together.

Our trip to Maine is coming up in June and Christine and I are looking forward to the relaxation and exploration of a state we'd never planned on visiting for vacation. I hear Acadia National Park is absolutely beautiful and Bar Harbor is a great place to stay. Plus I'll be in Stephen King country. I love that guy...sick mind and all.

CHECK THIS OUT!!!

The following essay was written by Christine's cousin Jessica before Christine's relapse. The words, like the message, paint a beautiful picture of how two young girls grew up as cousins and friends, and how a life changing event like Christine's leukemia affects more than just the person carrying the disease; everyone joins the fight. Please grab a box of tissues and enjoy. She's one hell of a writer:

An Essay, by Jessica Pierogowski

Chrissy was the pretty cousin. Actually, she was the perfect cousin. Although we were both blonde, I was blessed with bad eyes and crooked teeth, which required extremely thick bi-focal glasses and braces. Needless to say, I wasn't a very attractive eight-year-old. Chrissy, on the other hand, was the kind of girl who did everything right, from the time we were children and then directly on into her adult life. She was much quieter than me, except when she broke out into a fit of girly giggles, which would then set off my hoarse cackle. She was a great athlete-she played softball and her pitching skills eventually earned her a full scholarship to Long Island University. I was involved in dance classes, and although I showed talent and promise in that area, a perfect fouette turn in ballet class could not compare to pitching a perfect game, at least among our male cousins.

Chrissy and I each had our specific roles carved out for us from a very early age. These roles were illustrated in the ways we played as kids. Her Barbies' hair would be perfectly coifed, whereas the little amount my dolls had left on their heads was tinted blue from my mother's food coloring. She would be finishing her homework before the weekend started, while I decided to put my cousin's remote control car on top of my head and turn it on. My mother had to spend hours cutting that thing out of my hair.

My family still laughs about that at parties. She was the cousin who excelled and I was the oddball. It was only until last year that I realized what an important part these roles would play in our lives, and how fully she and I would come to rely on them.

Although we may have had every reason to be, Chrissy and I weren't competitive with one another. We were quite the opposite. We were the best of friends, and we rarely left each other's side. "Two peas in a pod" our mothers used to say. Both of our families lived in my Grandmother's apartment building, and we spent the time running up and down the stairs to play with one another. When we were about ten years old, my aunt and uncle decided to move to Staten Island to live with my aunt's mother. I was heartbroken. I went from seeing Chrissy every single day to the occasional holiday visit. While I focused on taking jazz and ballet in Greenpoint, she roughed it up with her softball pals an island away. We tried to reconnect during our visits, but at that point, we were moving in two different directions. As we went to different schools and delved into the world of boyfriends and makeup, we eventually grew apart. Even in our early adult lives Christine and I assumed our given roles. I moved out of my parents' home soon after high school to pursue my career in theater, while she went on to finish college with her Master's degree and find a job in her chosen field. While I was married and divorced in a year's time, she and her high school sweetheart of ten years, Tommy, had a fairy tale wedding. Soon after they wed they purchased a house they would renovate themselves, and were blessed with their first child, a beautiful baby girl named Kailey Anne. During the period following my divorce I pulled away from my family and focused on my career. This took a toll on my relationship with Chris. Although we were still cousins, the closeness we had shared as children was not the same. Things would soon take an unexpected and frightening turn. I would discover that the girl I played Barbies and rode Huffy bikes with had cancer. This discovery, and the effects of her disease, would catapult our relationship to a closer, more defined level. Our childhood roles were most important during this period, and, at times, would become reversed.

"What do you mean, an abnormality?"

I found out during a routine phone call made to my mother while on a break from French class that Christine found a lump in her breast while feeding Kailey. "After testing the lump, the doctors confirmed she had a blood disorder. Uncle Henry's going to call me with all the information when he gets home.

This was on Thursday. By Friday, she was diagnosed as having acute myeloid leukemia, admitted to MSKCC and was due to start chemotherapy that Monday. I couldn't believe this was happening. I hung up and realized that I would be conjugating irregular French verbs while my cousin was undergoing some painful test and I suddenly wanted very much to be near her. What I really wanted was for my mom to leap through that pay phone, hold me in her arms, and tell me my cousin was going to be all right. At that moment I was transformed into the eight year old with bifocals asking my mom why Chrissy was prettier than I was. In a heartbeat I would have donned those ugly glasses and crooked teeth if it would insure my cousin's safety.

On my first visit to Sloan Kettering I was filled with trepidation. "Will I cry when I see her? What will she look like?" Memories of our childhood filled my head as I waited for the elevator to take me to the 12th floor, home for leukemia patients. I had visions of me with my ice cream stained t-shirts and messy hair. Then I would think about Chrissy, who could pitch like a guy then take off her hat and her blond hair would come tumbling down, almost in slow motion like the girls in shampoo commercials. When I arrived at her room, I took a deep breath, and after securing my sterilized gown around my waist, I opened the door. I expected to see a pale, gaunt figure swallowed up by hospital blankets. In the room sitting up in bed was a cute girl in yellow pj's with a freshly buzzed blond head. The chemo had given her a slight dusting of freckles across her nose and cheeks, and although it sounds ridiculous even now, she had this glow about her. I walked in, smiled at Chrissy and noticed that she had a few partners in crime. Her husband, mother, and brother had buzzed their own heads to keep her company. At that moment, it wasn't so hard for me to understand why she was glowing.

A few minutes later, her nurse Desiree walked in. Desiree was a large black woman with an infectious laugh. The kind of laugh that begins with a howl and then flickers into giggles. She looked at Chris and said, "You remind me of someone, but I can't place who."

With a wry smile, Christine responded, "Yeah, I look like the Russian's wife in Rocky."

Desiree let out a howl, and soon the whole room was laughing. I looked at my cousin with amazement. Here is this girl, separated from her eight month old baby, filled with medication and IVs, and she's cracking jokes like a comedian. I stood there holding my perfectly baked chocolate chip cookies with my hair tied back to spare

Chrissy's feelings. During that first visit, I was just trying to do everything right, and she was just trying to make everyone laugh. In that moment I realized how much we had both grown up. We could easily switch out of our given roles to make them fit the situation at hand. Christine's choice was perfect because in a situation that was bigger than all of us, she managed to emerge victorious and continue to fight throughout her recovery.

I visited her several times during her two month stay at Sloan where I would come armed with cookies, magazines, and a variety of hats and scarves to cheer her spirits. It was during this time that I observed the greatest change in her. I watched her change from a delicate flower to a woman to be reckoned with. During the constant poking and prodding of her body, her spirit remained hopeful and she never lost her sense of humor. I watched a family and community rally around her. She was the girl everyone wanted to help. Her neighbors volunteered their time and money to furnish Tommy and Christine's new house with a much needed lawn and garden complete with a swing set for Kailey, as her mother organized a fundraising walk on Staten Island for leukemia. While collecting money for Fred's Team, a leukemia based charity connected with the New York City marathon, I realized I would never have been able to run those twenty-six point two miles without my cousin's example of courage and strength. Without ever knowing it, Christine brought out changes in all of us who were affected by her disease by focusing all her energy toward her recovery and not the leukemia itself. It was this positive outlook that took all of us outside of ourselves for a moment, and enabled us to become stronger individuals.

It has been a little over a year since Christine left the hospital and returned home. It is an unusually warm day for April, and I am sitting in the yard with her and Kailey. As we watch Kailey run around on her unsure little legs, there is an unspoken sense of closeness between us. It took a year of hospitals, baked goods, and phone calls filled with fearful updates to regain our childhood friendship. Christine is a wonderful wife and mother, and I remain the eccentric dreamer always running from one place to another. She's still perfect, and I 'm still a clown. We wouldn't have it any other way.

****

This update was a post-six month reality check. Now that the leukemia was gone, the emotional and psychological challenges were in full swing. Sometimes the scars you cannot see still run deep. The further we get past Day 0, the better it's supposed to get.

Day 192, Sunday, May 23, 2004:

Hello everyone. We are well past the six month mark and Christine is doing well. She was given a thumbs up from her doctor to do a few more things that she hadn't been able to do since the transplant. We were able to have our first BBQ and she's able to now do more things involving Kailey's care. Getting used to larger crowds is still something we need to work on though. It's very difficult to get comfortable in groups of 10 or more when we're not outside.

Although the six month mark was another huge step in the right direction, there's always the fear of getting sick and having to go back into the hospital. Christine wants to avoid that at all costs and sometimes it's very hard on her. I feel badly for her when she has a smile on her face for the benefit of those around her, but I know deep inside that she's a nervous wreck. She's trying so hard to fight the feelings of anxiety and, at times, despair. Sometimes I don't know what to do for her. I'll catch her sometimes staring out into space thinking, God only knows. It would be so nice if we could forget the whole thing happened, but in the back of her mind there's the little voice saying over and over again, "DON'T GET SICK!" It's the constant reminder that she spent months in the hospital over the last two plus years; the constant reminder of time away from our daughter.

It seems like day 100 was just yesterday, but on Memorial Day we'll already be at day 200!!! That is such an incredible thing to be able to write. Day 200 next Monday!!! I'm thrilled to be finishing this update on a positive note. Hopefully time will heal the wounds we cannot see.

****

Sometimes I was a little more excited than others, but as you can already tell it was for a very good reason. The baby steps seemed to be getting wider in stride and as low as the roller coaster could sometimes go, I sure as hell knew how to take advantage of the good feelings when it was riding high.

Day 198, Saturday, May 29, 2004:

Doesn't it seem like just yesterday we were hoping and praying for good old day-100, the first major milestone after Christine's blood counts began to come back after the transplant? It was 98 days ago. It's amazing that we're slowly making our way to day 200. Memorial Day, Monday May 31st is Day-200!!! I know I've mentioned it before, but it's worth mentioning again. Go ahead; say it out-loud, "day 200!" You didn't say it. Go on, a little louder so people look at you funny. Say it OUT-LOUD!!!! "DAY 200!!!!"

Going through the last seven or eight months with us through our ups and downs should make those words put a smile on your face. Not just a little smirk, or a "courtesy" smile, but a big old grandiose smile that says, "Heck! We're getting somewhere!" We're making ground and going full steam ahead and there's no looking back now. I see the end-zone and I've got the ball in a vice-grip and I'm not letting go...We're at the 5, the 10, the 20 the 35 we're across midfield...she could...go...all...the...way!

Christine had her six month bone marrow biopsy this week. The last one showed her bone marrow to be 100% donor and there weren't any signs of leukemia. We're looking for the same results this time around. We'll get the results in about a month. She also finished what could be her last treatment of IVIG. This was the drug that was boosting her immune system until she could make her own. In one month she'll take a blood test to determine whether she needs additional doses, but at 6 months out she should be making enough on her own. We're very happy to not have another doctor appointment for a while.

Our trip to Maine is quickly approaching and we cannot wait to go away to do nothing. This will be our first vacation for R&R in some time.

Christine and I had 3 BBQs lined up for this weekend but we haven't decided if we're going to make them all or whether it will be too much for her. We still have to make sure she doesn't overdo it. Her stamina is much better and she does not get very tired until the evening. This week she gave Kailey a bath and will continue to do so every now and then.

Christine's dad, who had been coming to our house at 7:30AM since she came home from the hospital pushed arrival time back to 10AM this week. She's beginning to take back a little more of her regular responsibilities. Christine's mom still comes by to help her at about noon and stays until about 4PM, and then Chrissy picks back up again, doing more of the things she was able to do before the relapse. I'm extremely proud of her; taking back a little more of her life from the cancer that tried to take it away. I see the fight in her eyes every day. She amazes me.

I caught Christine reading back through some of the older website entries on the archive pages yesterday. Together, we looked back on many of the stories captured in writing. We laughed, cried, and remembered how far she's come...

Before I go, please do me one favor; tell someone close to you that you love them. It's funny how often we take for granted the time we spend with someone we love without actually saying those three very important words. Even if they know it already, say it anyway.

****

As I've mentioned, many people were involved in helping to fight leukemia and other blood disorders. Christine's support network ran so wide that even her alma mater joined the fight. So many wonderful pieces of news in this regard started rolling in that I did my best spread the word.

Day 201, Tuesday, June 1, 2004:

EXTRA! EXTRA! READ ALL ABOUT IT!!! ST. JOHN VILLA AND ST. PETER'S BOYS HIGH SCHOOL RAISE $10,000 IN THE FIGHT AGAINST LEUKEMIA!!!

You may have read it in the Advance [our local paper] a month or so back, but the story is here again. The combined high schools of Christine's alma mater and her brother's alma mater came together to raise $10,000 for the Leukemia & Lymphoma Society. They presented the check to Christine this evening as a donation to the "Angels for Christine" Light The Night team.

The Villa student council was on-hand to present Christine the check at their closing dinner. Christine was joined by me, Kailey, Christine's mom and dad and members of the LLS. We are proud and feel so honored to be a part of such an amazing school. Christine held back tears as she stood in front of the student council to thank them for their generosity and hard work.

We also would like to thank all the students of both schools for holding such a wonderful event for such a worthy cause. Some of you may not realize the lives you've touched by putting together such a generous donation. You've touched our hearts and shown that as the leaders of tomorrow you can set out to accomplish great things. To the seniors, good luck with your future endeavors, and for the underclassman, it's great to have you back next year.

All our love,
The Wonicas

****

We finally went on our first family vacation since the transplant. We took a trip to Maine. From a hospital bed in isolation to a family vacation in Maine in just 230 short days. Isn't life great!

Day 231, Thursday, July 1, 2004:

Hear ye, hear ye. It has been a few weeks since I last wrote to tell you of Christine's progress, but progress is a great word for it. Today is day 231!!! I cannot believe that we are 31 days past the 200 day mark. Everyone knows that November 13th will be one year post transplant, which means we're quickly approaching the eight-month mark (July 13th.) It wasn't long ago, a couple of weeks to be exact, that Christine, Kailey and I ventured to the middle of Maine to take in a breathtaking part of the US that we previously had never seen. We went to Bar Harbor, ME, roughly a ten-hour drive from Staten Island. We split the trip up by book-ending the five-day Maine stay with short visits to my sister's home in Rhode Island. The whole trip was a wonderful experience. Our room at the Bar Harbor Inn was right on the water and our balcony looked out over the harbor's three or so islands that were close to the shoreline. We spent a great deal of time relaxing and doing a whole lot of nothing, but we did manage to learn a few things about Maine. Maine is well known for a few specific things: moose, blueberries, maple syrup, and lobsters. Christine had her allowance of one lobster but saved it for the last day of our trip. She feasted on a two-pounder that melted in her mouth. We didn't see any moose, but I did feast on some of the best blueberry pancakes I've ever had. They were delightful, especially with the local maple syrup!

Kailey Anne made some friends while on the trip and played a lot by the swingset. She's a character and a half. Without even knowing the kids at the Inn, she was already telling us she wanted to go out and play with her "friends." It wasn't long before she worked her way into their games of hide and seek, tag, "Pokemon", singing, dancing, and getting dirty. It was nice to see her out there with other children her own age.

Very close to our location in Maine was the Acadia National Park. We spent some time driving through the park and thoroughly enjoyed the beauty of the scenery. It is simply amazing how natural some pieces of the U.S. can look after living so close to the big city. It's almost like a tall glass of water after a long run. You can even smell the purity in the air and almost hear your lungs say, "Give me more of that!!!" The park was amazing and we did some sightseeing, picture taking and a little hiking.

All in all, it was a vacation that we needed more than we knew. It was relaxing. It was just the three of us for the first time in a long time and we enjoyed it very much. We experienced a little bit more of what life is all about.

Unfortunately, when we returned home from Maine it was right back to medical business. Christine had her third of six necessary spinal taps a couple of weeks ago and it went fairly well. We noticed she has to eat very light after the spinal tap due to her nerves and the effect they have on her stomach. She is tentatively done with the IVIG and 100% complete with the Rituxan. She's still taking some of the pilled medication. Chrissy is getting out and about and handling social gatherings a little better, but still easing into bigger events. Small venues of 5-10 are preferred over larger turnouts. We're still taking it one day at a time.

Thanks:

I would like to thank all of you for continuing to stick by us as we fight day in and day out to take back our life from this horrible disease. We're finally enjoying our home, our family, and our time together a lot more than in the previous 2+ years. I cannot express the gratitude I feel knowing so many of you are behind us praying in the background. We never forget the strength you help us keep and the influence you've had on our individual and familial survival. We are truly blessed.

****

Looking to give back to some of the people who helped us has been a big part of our continued fight. We strive to make a difference against blood cancers. As Christine made progress, the updates became less frequent as we focused a little more on just being a family.

Day 260, Friday, July 30, 2004:

Although "no news is GREAT news," I know it's been a while since the last update so let's get to it....

Christine continues to do very well after a full week of very bad headaches and a few days of vomiting because of the latest spinal tap. The doctors used the "large" needle due to scar tissue around the area from previous lumbar punctures. We know from past experience that the large needle doesn't work well for Christine so we have to make sure that during the next and final 2 spinal taps that they scrap the large needle and stick with the smaller one. This was Christine's 4th spinal tap in as many months. She has two more to go and then that part of the treatment is complete. (As I've mentioned before, they pull some spinal fluid to verify there aren't any leukemia cells in the nervous system. Then they inject some chemotherapy into her spinal cord just in case there's anything hiding in there.)

Chrissy continues to get better each day and as we approach the nine month mark her spirits are high and the fight in her is still very strong. Kailey's birthday is coming up on August 3rd and she's turning three years old. Christine and I are throwing a party for her with all her little friends and cousins.

Christine and I have been busy with the house and family outings. Except for a rough week with the spinal tap, we have had something to do each and every weekend this summer. It's nice to stay busy and spend more time with family and friends.

Light The Night

Last week was a big week for Kailey and me as we gave a speech at the kick-off dinner for this year's Light The Night walk sponsored by The Leukemia & Lymphoma Society.

This is the third year that "Angels for Christine" will be walking in the event. This year, Christine will have the honor of walking with a white balloon, signifying she's a survivor.

Kailey experienced her first public speaking event at the kick-off dinner and stole the show. I stood there on the podium in front of 400+ people and began to recount our story and the need for support and Kailey was in perfect form. She waved to the crowd twice as I adjusted the microphone and the crowd laughed both times. Then, as I spoke, she interrupted me twice by saying, "Dad, is it my turn to talk now?" I replied, "Not yet honey." (Again the crowd laughed each time). When I made the mistake of ignoring her the third time, she grabbed me by the face and pulled my head toward her and asked, "My turn now?" (again, laughter). It was a great setting and a great event setup very nicely by the LLS staff. It was the kind of event that makes you happy to be a part of such a wonderful team of people. The finale came as I said thank you to the crowd. I put Kailey close enough to the microphone to speak into it and she let out a rather loud "Thank you" of her own. The crowd laughed again. I think we'll take our show in the road:-)

The best part about getting to speak in front of the crowd was getting to tell a small part of my wife's story. I continue to be the proud husband of a fighter; a woman looking a life altering event straight in the eye and saying, "You're not going to beat me." She's amazing.

Updates

There are a number of updates to give and some congratulations to some very special people in our lives:

I'M GOING TO BE AN UNCLE! Congrats to my brother Scott!!! Pretty soon, a cousin for Kailey!!! [Little Scott was born, and they added Ryan and Matty.]

Remember to keep November 13th, Christine's one year mark, open on your calendars. It looks like we'll be having a party at our house and you're all invited to celebrate with us!

****

Anniversaries tend to remind us of what we've been through and how far we've come. Just as we celebrate Christine's new birthday on November 13th, we tend to feel somber on the days that remind us of her initial diagnosis or when we received the call that she'd relapsed.

<u>Day 285, Tuesday, August 24, 2004:</u>

Kailey turned three on August 3rd. We had a small party with a bunch of her friends and their families. It was a great time and a lot of fun. It was nice to see her blow out the candles, open her own gifts with enthusiasm and say, "thank you" for each one. Kailey turning three has been the highlight of a very nice summer; a summer of healing and praying.

Every so often I get the feeling that none of it ever happened, that I fell asleep and had a nightmare. I forget about the hours, days, weeks and months in the hospital, praying my wife would recover quickly. But then it comes back and I remember staring at the clock, willing time to move faster so her wounds would heal. I remember the countless prayers and talks with God, asking him to make her better. "Let it go away and never come back." Then, just like that I'm singing happy birthday to my daughter and watching the kids at the party fight for a spot closest to the cake. I'm sitting and watching Carmini the Clown make us all laugh by pulling flowers out of an empty bag and making a rabbit appear as if from thin air. At that moment the world is back to normal and everything makes sense; at least for a little while.

Just over a year ago Christine, Kailey and I went on vacation to Wildwood Crest. We had a time to remember. While we were there, the blackout of 2003 hit NYC, but our lights stayed on. It was perfect timing…and then we came home. Our return is what keeps me up at night. Like a bad movie it replays in my mind over and over. It's what wakes me up from a deep sleep to check on my wife and baby. It's the nightmare I can't escape. It's a point in time that makes me want to curl up into a ball and sleep until the "boogeyman" goes away. Unfortunately, it's the monster in the closet you have to face before you can go on with the rest of your life. The day I found that my wife had relapsed is a day I will always remember, though I long to forget. The one year anniversary of that day is tough to get through.

As Christine prepares for a bone marrow biopsy on Wednesday, I think to myself, "It must be getting easier." Then I'll walk into a room and find her lost in thought, an expressionless look upon her face. I've known Christine long enough to know exactly what she's thinking, and my heart breaks. I've spoken to her about what she's feeling. She says that 90% of the time everything's fine. It's the 10% that takes her to another place. It's that 10% that breaks her down sometimes. The important part is that she builds herself right back up. At one point that 10% of time she was in a bad place was closer to 100%. It's worked its way down and I hope it keeps on going. Pretty soon the 10% may be 5% and then 3% and then 1%. It may even make it lower than that. The unfortunate thing is that it will probably never hit zero. At times like these however, Christine can turn to her family and friends to pull her through.

It's Day 283 and the anniversary of a very difficult time in our lives. As we make it through, let's keep our sights on the very special time quickly approaching. November 13th. It may sound biblical when I say it, but it is true. It was the day Christine was given new life.

****

Finally, a spinal tap that didn't make Christine feel badly.

Day 301, Thursday, September 9, 2004:

Two new items have come up since I last wrote. Christine has completed her 5th spinal tap and has only one more to go! She received the spinal tap yesterday on day 300!!! Yes, we have reached day 300 and that means we are getting very close to that oh-so-special one-year mark on November 13th.

The spinal tap went so much better than the last one. Christine and I explained the need for the smaller needle to be used in the procedure because of the excruciating headaches she suffers when the larger needle was used. The radiologist relayed the message to the doctor who performed the best spinal tap Christine has received to date. Additionally, the doctor was so pleasant to work with that we hope Christine will get her again the next time. Unfortunately, you can't request the spinal tap doctors like you can a regular physician because they're on some sort of rotation between buildings, but you can bet we're going to try.

Thanks to everyone for keeping up to date on Christine's progress.

****

I still don't like to talk much about the initial research I conducted when Christine was preparing for her bone marrow transplant. Sure, I would filter out some of the harsh details, but that didn't mean they didn't weigh heavily on me at times. After Christine's relapse, the bone marrow transplant was the legitimate "plan B," and the best chance we had at saving Christine's life. We knew that. So it didn't matter that the chance of surviving a bone marrow transplant in 2003 was 30-50%. WHAT?! Yes, only 30-50%. When I first read that I searched and searched to try and find documentation that told me she had a better chance. I could not, so I stopped reading. The big difference as I wrote this next update was that it was no longer November 13, 2003. It was NOVEMBER 13, 2004, CHRISTINE'S NEW 1st BIRTHDAY!!!!

Christine's new 1st birthday was one of the greatest days ever. We celebrated with a few hundred of our family and friends. We actually threw two separate parties that day, one at the same hall where we had our wedding reception, the Staaten on Staten Island, and then at our home "open house" style. We couldn't wait for that day to get here and then we didn't want it to end. People came from all over the country to spend that special day with us. It was absolutely amazing!

One Year Mark! November 13, 2004:

We are very happy we were able to spend Christine's one-year post transplant day with many of you. We'd like to thank you all for the thoughtful cards and gifts. Christine's smile was plastered on her face right up until the moment she hit the pillow. It was an amazing day in which we renewed our vows in front of our family and friends and watched and listened as Christine gave a speech that brought tears to everyone's eyes. It was utterly amazing. I have a very special woman.

Christine's cousin Theresa surprised her by flying in from Nebraska. Theresa bought the plane ticket over 3 months ago and we kept it a good secret for a long time. It was so fitting to have her with us. She and Christine write and talk often. They were very close growing up. Having her here made the day even more special.

Aunt Leona made it in from Arizona too. It was so nice to have her with us. She has been such a big supporter that it wouldn't have been the same without her. We all went out to breakfast the morning after the party.

Christine and the Doctor

Christine has had her last spinal tap, her one-year bone marrow biopsy and only requires 2 immunizations because the other antibodies already appear in her blood, which is still 100% the donor's.

Christine's immune system is coming back better than even her doctor had expected and the surprise has been a pleasant one. Christine is getting over her first cold since her transplant and has shown that her body is able to fight. We're all very happy about her progress and even happier that her doctor visits are getting further and further apart. Her next bone marrow biopsy isn't for another six months. It's not long before Christine can stop all her medications and feast on the two things she's been craving most; sushi and a Big Mac (but not at the same meal!)

Our family took an awesome two week trip to Florida. We drove down and back to avoid the airplane's circulated air. We had an amazing time. Kailey was a champ the whole 16+ hours there and back. Her only complaints came during the last 3 hours of the trip when she decided it was a good time to tell me, "Dad, this is taking too long."

We spent a few days in St. Augustine, a few in Universal Studio's Royal Pacific Resort, a few days in Boynton Beach with Christine's Aunt Bernadette and the last 5 days at the Caribbean Beach Resort in Walt Disney World. The trip was a long time coming and Christine deserved every second of it. It was Christine and Kailey's first time in Disney and it was most definitely a magical experience.

****

Over a year after donating his stem cells for Christine's transplant, the donor entered our world once again. It had been so long since we received the letter from him in the hospital room just before the transplant. It was the last time we would hear anything about him, until now.

1 year and 10 days, November 22, 2004:

I haven't written much about the donor in the updates because we don't know anything about him other than he's a male with ten of the ten major chromosomes in his white blood cells matching Christine's and he agreed to donate some of his stem cells to save her life. There are strict guidelines for donating bone marrow or stem cells and not being given any information about the donor is just one of them. We weren't even allowed to know his name until at least a year post transplant. I'm sure there are many good reasons for all the rules given everything that can go wrong during a BMT. For example, how would someone react if a donor's blood failed to save the patient? Would the patient's family blame the donor? Since things like that can easily happen, I'm sure it has a lot to do with the strict policies. Even after a year there was no guarantee we would ever get to know more about Christine's bone marrow [stem cell] donor. All the chips would have to fall into place. So you can imagine our excitement to find out he was willing to exchange information with us.

Our donor is a 39-year-old man named Robert Browning. The funny thing is we were very close to his hometown while we were in Florida recently. We found out about Robert after we returned from our vacation. He is from the Tampa area! We communicated with Robert, our hero, through the blood donation centers of MSKCC and the Donor Center in Florida. He, unfortunately, wasn't able to make it to the one year celebration due to work responsibilities but there is some GREAT news; his company may fly us down to meet him for the first time. We can't wait to finally say "thank you" in person or even get the chance to speak with him on the phone. I can't even imagine how emotional that day will be. Thank you again Robert from Florida!!!!

It's getting kind of late so I'm going to wrap it up for this evening. As Thanksgiving approaches, I think back to last year's celebration. I was thanking God that my wife was still alive as we sat in her hospital room on the 11th floor of MSKCC, the transplant floor. Christine didn't get to see Kailey that day.

It's just one year later and it's amazing how drastically things can change. It's safe to say that this year, like every year to come, we will enjoy Thanksgiving just a little bit more than we used to. We have a lot to be thankful for.

****

This update captures an amazing day in our lives. A day forever etched in our hearts as a family with a hero.

<u>1 year 13 days, Thursday, November 25 2004, Thanksgiving Day:</u>

Hello everyone and Happy Thanksgiving. Christine and I wanted to get a great big "Happy Turkey Day" out to all our friends and family before the day was over. The day just wouldn't be complete without it. We had an amazing day today.

First of all, I never thought of waking up in my own bed with Christine as a privilege, but that's exactly how it felt. It was so nice to get up, have a cup of coffee and watch the parade with my family. Kailey had her 'warm chocolate milk' and Christine and I had our coffee as we watched the floats and balloons parade down the streets of Manhattan from the comfort of our living room couch. Then Santa came (in the parade) and we danced to Christmas carols on the living room rug, a tradition we missed last year and settled for Kailey and I dancing with Christine over a webcam.

After a while Chrissy broke off to get ready for dinner at her parents' house and Kailey and I continued to dance; right up until the clock told me we better get a move on.

The morning was even better than that though. This morning we spoke, for the first time, to our hero in Florida. This morning we spoke to Robert, the 39 year old volunteer, who donated his bone marrow so Christine could start fresh. While I spoke to this soft-spoken gentleman from the Tampa area, I was not amazed at all at how nice he was. I was not shocked by his gentle heart and modesty. As I thanked him for the role he played in saving Christine he simply said, "It is what anyone with a decent heart would do for someone in need." Talk about downplaying his role.

I spoke with Robert for almost 35 minutes before Christine had gained some composure to speak on the phone. (Now I know why she wanted me to speak first.) As soon as I said, "Hello Robert, my name is Tom Wonica and I've been looking forward to speaking with you for a little over a year now," she was balling. Sitting right next to me on the couch, my wife was crying tears of joy knowing she was about to actually speak with her bone marrow donor for the first time.

It took a long conversation before Christine was alright to speak, but I enjoyed every second of it; and then, the time came. She said hello to her hero, and the tears came again, but she was able to speak through them. She told him how much he meant to her and our family. She told him how grateful she was for all he had done. He continued to be modest, but Christine made it clear....he was now a part of our family.

Robert told Christine how much he'd been looking forward to speaking with her. She told him how much speaking to him on Thanksgiving meant to her. They spoke for about half an hour and then said goodbye, wishing our family a Happy Thanksgiving. A lot was said in the 65 minutes we were all on the phone. There were some interesting coincidences discussed in our conversations:

1) Robert's birthday is July 24th which is our wedding anniversary,

2) The man loves football...I love football. (Bucs fan or not, he is a diehard...woooo whooo!

3) His wife has family in Jersey City and they visit every so often so we may get to see him and his family when they make the trip.

4) Robert's wife is Polish and Christine and I both have strong Polish lineage.

5) Robert's older daughter just joined softball. Christine can definitely give her some pointers.

…and the most amazing…

6) Robert donated blood one day out of the blue because he saw a blood donation bus outside his church after mass. After the donation they asked him if he'd like to be on the national bone marrow registry and he said yes. THIS WASN'T LONG BEFORE CHRISTINE'S INITIAL DIAGNOSIS! Robert's simple answer, "yes," coupled with the bus, church and Robert being there saved Christine; divine intervention at work.

Christine, Kailey and I will be planning our trip to Florida to hopefully meet Robert and his family before the holidays. He was such a nice guy we can't wait to spend some more time getting to know him and his family.

Before I sign off for the evening I'd like to once again thank you all for your love and support as we continue our fight. This Thanksgiving night we send our thanks. I'd like to send a very special thanks to some very special people:

Robert, Lisa, Robert II, Brittany, and Morgan….thank you from the bottom of our hearts and God bless you all.

Happy Thanksgiving!

****

Getting to finally talk to our hero was an amazing moment in our lives. Getting to actually speak with the person who, simply through the goodness of his heart, put himself out there "just in case" he could help someone was like a dream come true. This man put his life on hold to save a total stranger. If there was ever an example of a person living his beliefs; living in the image of his faith, Robert Browning is that example. It was such a special occasion for our family that words cannot do it justice. If only we could get the chance to actually meet this wonderful man in person. If only we had the opportunity to shake his hand like a friend and hug him like a brother. If only we could look him in the eyes so he could see exactly how much what he did meant to us; how much he now meant to us. Enter Florida Blood Services, the blood collection center that collected Robert's blood donation that led to him being on the national bone marrow registry. It seems the list of heroes just got a bit longer.

Chapter 10

The Hero, Robert Browning

One of the final entries in the Care for Christine Support network "journal" documents an incredibly special moment in Christine's journey. Metaphorically, it highlights one of the brightest lights at the end of the tunnel; a catalyst that has helped Christine along the long road of healing that would still lie ahead. Robert Browning of Tampa Florida, wherever you are at this very moment, I want every person reading this book to know just how incredible you are as a human being. You are a perfect example of selflessness. My brother, you walked the walk and continue to do so every day. We need more people in the world like you. You more than deserve a chapter with your name on it!!

<u>1 year and 30 Days, December 12, 2004:</u>

The humidity was thick in the air as we arrived at Tampa Airport on Thursday night (12/9/2004). We enjoyed the trip from NY's JFK, flying on Jet Blue. It was a nice plane ride. Although Christine was nervous about the flight, there were other things on her mind. What would the first meeting with her donor be like? It seemed surreal, a word which describes most of our last three years. Christine's parents were at the airport to see us off as we headed toward a meeting with this very special man and his very special family.

We landed in Tampa at roughly 10:05PM and made our way to the baggage claim. As we approached, we saw a man holding up a sign which read "Welcome to Tampa, Christine, Tom, and Kailey Wonica." The man holding the sign was Ivan, an employee with Florida Blood Services, another group of heroes. He was there to drive us to the hotel where we would spend the next two nights. Ivan was a happy man with a big heart. He made us feel welcomed and his smile told us he enjoyed what he did. Part of his job was helping to save lives.

Ivan treated Christine like she was a celebrity. "Everyone's been talking about your arrival for some time. We all couldn't wait to meet you." By the time we had gotten the luggage and arrived at the hotel we felt as if Ivan were an old time friend. We'd experience that a lot on this trip. There was definitely a magic in the air this Florida night and we weren't even in Disney.

We arrived at the hotel by 10:45PM, and were checked into our room, room 615. Ivan said good night and we made plans to be picked up at 8:15AM the next morning (12/10) to begin the day's events.

Christine, Kailey and I went up to the room and ordered a Domino's pizza (not the best idea) and then went to bed. It was difficult to fall asleep right away. The excitement and anticipation was building. Tomorrow was the day.

We awoke at 6:45AM and began getting ready. It didn't take a cup of coffee to get Christine moving this morning. The anticipation was doing a fine job all its own. We met Ivan downstairs at 8:15AM and had breakfast in the hotel restaurant. At breakfast we spoke with Ivan about the day's plans. Christine spoke of how nervous she was to speak in front of the planned reunion, where she would meet Robert Browning for the first time. Ivan offered encouragement, but Christine and I had worked out a plan. If she got stuck she would let me know and I'd help her out. She was too nervous to prepare a speech so I didn't know what to expect. I prayed she wouldn't faint.

We arrived at the Teco Peoples Gas facility at roughly 9:15AM. We were 45 minutes early. When we arrived, Ivan called Katrina Holley on his mobile phone. Katrina is the Program Director of the Florida Blood Services' Marrow Donor

Program. She was nervous that Ivan had gotten us there too early since our transport vehicle had the Florida Blood Services' logo on the van. She didn't want us to attract the media before the reunion. She was afraid they would "swarm" the van. At hearing this, Christine couldn't believe it. "Swarm?" she thought. The anticipation grew.

Ivan left the Teco parking lot and we drove around historic Ybor, an area of Tampa being restored around its early Latin American heritage. Ivan gave us the tour.

On our way around the town, we spotted one of the 18 blood donation buses that Florida Blood Services owns [at the time of this writing]. It is one of 18 buses that must collect 600-750 pints of blood a day to support the Tampa area's needs. It was one of those buses that was outside Robert Browning's church the day he decided to donate a pint of blood to "help someone out."

"Would you like to join the National Bone Marrow Registry Mr. Browning?"

"Sure, why not."

At roughly 10 minutes to 10AM we got the call from Katrina to head back to the Teco Peoples Gas offices where Robert's company had offered to hold the reunion. The ceremony was already underway when Christine was brought through a side door undetected. Kailey and I were right by her side. Ivan's partner, Glorea "the transporter" led the way. Glorea had delivered Robert's stem cells to MSKCC on November 13, 2003. That same night they were given to Christine so she could begin her road to recovery.

Once in the building we waited in a hallway outside the conference room where Robert was speaking in front of the gathered crowd of just over 100 reporters, cameramen, Teco employees, friends, members of the Tampa chapter of The Leukemia & Lymphoma Society, members of Florida Blood Services and others. His wife Lisa was by his side. "The happiest day of my life, besides marrying my wife…and my three kids, was getting that call on Thanksgiving morning and finding out that [Christine] was alright."

Robert broke down more than once while speaking that day, his emotions as strong as his heart. After Robert had said a few words, Katrina spoke a few as well. When she was finished she announced Christine's name.

Silence fell across the room as we made our way toward the door leading to the conference room. There was a lump in my throat the size of an apple as I followed my wife who had Kailey by the hand. As we entered, the silence broke with the sound of applause. We entered the room and passed by the chairs and the podium and Christine and Robert embraced for the first time, finally face to face. Excitement flooded my heart as tears flooded almost every eye in the room. The news cameras were focused in on the hero and the survivor; the hope and the inspiration. Kailey and I hugged Robert next, and again a dreamlike feeling overcame me. Here he was…our new brother; our angel.

The next half an hour was a whirlwind of emotion. Christine spoke in front of the crowd and delivered an incredible thanks to everyone in the room. She gave account of her struggles and her fight with leukemia; of her need to beat this disease for her daughter and her family; of her thanks to Robert for saving her family and her life. It was a wonderful, heartfelt moment for everyone to cherish before Robert, again with tears in his eyes, stood to hug the woman he saved. I said a few words of thanks and then Katrina stood to speak about the importance of donating blood and being added to the national bone marrow registry. She spoke about the wonder of saving someone's life; something we now know so well.

The ceremony was followed by interviews with the media. ABC, NBC, and CBS were all present with their local affiliates. The Tampa Tribune was also there covering for the Saturday edition. Christine found herself surrounded by four cameras and a microphone as a reporter asked questions about her experience with leukemia and being a recipient of a bone marrow donation. She answered the questions with the composure of an actress and the smile of an angel. When she was done we enjoyed refreshments offered by Teco and spoke with some of Robert's colleagues. They confirmed what we already knew; that Robert is a very special individual and is loved by everyone who knows him.

Robert's character and big heart are something his entire family shares. His lovely wife Lisa, their beautiful daughters Brittany (11 yrs) and Morgan (6 yrs), and Big lil' Man Robert II (12 yrs) were such a pleasure to spend time with. We went to dinner with Robert, his family and members of the Florida Blood Services' staff that night. It was a great chance to spend even more time together.

Kailey had such a wonderful time with the Browning children I felt like we were with family. We spent a great deal of time talking about how special the weekend was and how amazing an experience it was to finally meet them all. We spoke about getting together again in the near future; and how we hope a long-standing friendship grows out of our meeting.

The next day Florida Blood Services treated us and the Brownings to a day at the Florida Aquarium. It was a pleasure to walk around the aquarium and get to know each other a little more. We had lunch later that day and then the Brownings took us for a ride around the Tampa area to show us the sites. It was great to sit back and enjoy the ride before heading back to the airport. Robert and his family saw us off at the airport, his family running to the window to wave goodbye as the shuttle took us from the baggage area to the security gate. We waved back; and then we cried. We miss the Brownings. We're thankful we had the chance to finally meet Robert and his family, but two days were definitely not enough.

Words cannot describe how wonderful they were. Robert's heart of gold is evident in everything he does. His wife's love and support were clear and her kindness radiating. His kids were an amazing trio of love, fun, and respect for life, all clear in the smiles on their faces. We look forward to seeing them again very soon. This was a friendship created in heaven and strengthened by the wind of angels' wings. There's not much more I can say to express how deep our feelings run. So I'll leave it at that.

There are so many heroes in Christine's story. We've heard about our friends and family at home and the doctors and nurses who helped make Christine better, but there are so many players. Christine's recovery is like a recipe of people and events. The recipe is not something you can quite capture on paper, but something that gets mixed together and in the end you hope and pray that the cake rises.

God bless the Brownings and their big hearts. God bless Robert's blood.

Thanks and God bless Teco Peoples Gas for seeing the good in what Robert did, and for holding the gift of life so close to their hearts.

Thanks to the management staff at Teco [at the time of this writing] for making it easy for Robert to give of himself,

Thanks to his colleagues and friends for their support of Robert. We love the messages you've sent confirming what we already know; that he's an angel on earth.

Thanks to Katrina, Ivan, Robert and the rest of the Marrow Donor Program team at Florida Blood Services for all you do.

Thanks to Florida Blood Services for having such an incredible program and for keeping up the fight.

Thanks to the Tampa news stations and newspapers that covered this event.

Spreading the word is how we can save more lives.

Thanks to you all for reading my updates, regardless of how long or how confusing they are. Telling you our story is my goal. Meeting Robert and his family completes one BIG chapter in Christine's road to recovery. Thank you for sharing it with us.

Christine's message to Robert during our trip says it all. I leave you with the words she delivered to her hero at the press conference:

> I've thought often about my life and where I am today.
> I've thought back to the day I found out I had
> > leukemia…and the day I found it had come back.
> I've thought back to the fear and the anxiety that swept
> > through me as I fought hard to defeat this disease with
> > an unknown hero by my side.
> I've thought back to what may have been if not for you.
> Thank you for taking the time to help someone in need.
> Thank you for taking the time to donate blood.
> Thank you for joining the bone marrow registry.
> Thank you for saving my family.
> Thank you for saving my life.
>
> ~Christine Wonica

With Christine's words to Robert, her hero, still fresh in our minds, it is with pride and a warm heart that I say "good night." We will all sleep very well tonight.

****

Chapter 11

Closure

It was November 12, 2008, just one day before Christine's official cure date; almost five years since her BMT and over six years since her first diagnosis with leukemia. We waited impatiently in the lobby of Suite 4 at MSKCC waiting for her doctor to arrive.

We pulled into the parking lot early that morning for the 8AM doctor's visit. Christine had barely slept the night before, her mind and body filled with anticipation. We followed our usual ritual. Christine's parents arrived at our house at 6:45AM for the drive into the city, while my mom arrived at our house at the same time to take care of Kailey's morning routine of getting dressed and off to school on time. Christine's brother was with us too for this trip; he would make a blood donation at MSKCC as we went in for this monumental check-up.

Christine had already made her contribution of blood which now stood in a host of vials for the morning's tests when the doctor walked past us in the waiting room. As "good morning" left her lips I could feel the already tense atmosphere tighten even further. Most of that tension came directly from the seat to my right, where Christine sat. She smiled at me through clenched teeth, her legs rocking back and forth in a steady nervous rhythm all the while.

It wasn't long after the doctor passed us in the waiting room that one of the assistants came to show us to our destiny; the third room on the right. One by one we filed into the room and assumed our positions. Christine hopped up onto the examination table and we took our places in the seats surrounding her as we had done too many times before. We each prayed to ourselves that the news would be good. We prayed that Christine's blood counts were still in the normal ranges; that the leukemia was gone for good.

We all knew that although November 13th was Christine's official five-year mark, it was the results of this morning's tests that would determine whether that day would be one of the happiest days of our lives or the beginning of yet another tough journey. Just the possibility of bad news brought a shiver down my spine as I tried hard to focus only on happy thoughts.

After roughly five minutes of agonizingly nervous small talk, the doorknob rattled and turned. The door swung open and in walked the doctor, a piece of paper in hand. She extended it toward Christine.

"Congratulations Christine. Everything is normal. You did it!"

We sat still for a split second, processing the words that just rolled off the doctor's tongue; those sweet sounding words that just told us, Christine was CURED!!!

Our reactions were a mixture of triumphant cheering and emotionally charged laughter. There were tears mixed in with the excitement that turned to smiles and then back to tears in an instant. I jumped up and the doctor handed me the paper that held the results of the morning's blood work just so I could see it with my very own eyes. At that moment, it was the sweetest, most precious thing I had ever seen in my whole life!

Christine and I hugged and kissed right there in the doctor's office. We looked into each other's eyes and smiled. The moment was magical, like so many others we'd shared and experienced on our long journey to cure Christine.

Right there, at that moment, a weight of unimaginable size was lifted from Christine's back. She was practically floating as we continued on to our celebratory breakfast at the Starlight Diner, just as we had done after every successful doctor appointment over the previous 5 years. That evening we had dinner with some of our closest friends and although the official day was still a night's sleep away, it was a celebration none the less.

On the morning of November 13th I took off from work to be with my wife on her special day. We awoke with smiles that stayed on our faces until we fell asleep that night. We spent most of the time sitting and hugging, laughing and talking, on the couch in the living room of our home. As I write this, most of that day seems like a dream; a glorious, remarkable dream. We dropped off and picked up Kailey from school together. We continued the rest of the day in the same way, as a family.

That evening, we had dinner at the same local Italian restaurant we'd eaten at each of the previous four years on November 13th. This time, our family was with us. During dinner we toasted Christine's health and recovery. We honored the work of the doctors and nurses, her donor Robert Browning and his family, and all those who helped us make it through the tough times. We especially remembered the Care for Christine Support Network and the special people who traveled the journey with us through our website and updates. The final update was posted that evening and can still be found at http://CareforChristine.com.

It was most definitely a long and trying road to that family dinner. Christine had gone through more than anyone should have to in their life. She was forced down a road less traveled and made it through to the other side, and we traveled it with her.

As I look back on the years that leukemia has taken from our family I am not bitter or angry, but grateful. Not everybody will get to travel to there and back again on the wings of hope and heroes in their lifetime; but we were chosen. Looking back I can say without pause that it was a tough road for my wife and for us as a family, but when you make it successfully to the end of the journey, there's no better feeling in the entire world.

****

It was sometime after Christine's one-year post-transplant milestone when she, Kailey and I got in our car and passed through the EZ-Pass lane of the New Jersey turnpike and began a new drive down I-95. We stopped only for food and rest until we reached Florida. As I looked around at the smiles on Christine and Kailey's faces I knew we had both been right. We needed to get away, but Christine needed to get better first. From my point of view, I couldn't have asked for anything more.

Author's note to Christine

To My Wife Christine,

It's fitting that these final words close a chapter in our lives; to be replaced with memories of happier, more cheerful times together as a family. But no matter how far away this time in our life gets, I will never forget the story of the survivor who journeyed to there and back again on the wings of Hope and Heroes. I will never forget the courage and determination of one very special young woman. A woman I'm proud to call my wife.

You're cured!

I love you,
Tommy

CARE FOR CHRISTINE SUPPORT NETWORK

If Christine's story has inspired you, there are a number of links below to help you get more involved in fighting blood cancer. Especially check out the fantastic programs offered by the Leukemia and Lymphoma Society (LLS). Another great way to help is to donate blood and get added to the bone marrow registry. Should they call you as a match for someone, please say "Yes." You could be the next Robert Browning, helping another mom get home to her baby.

You can also visit http://CareforChristine.com to make a donation to the LLS through our walk team, Angels for Christine. Just follow the links.

RELEVANT, USEFUL AND FUN LINKS

Care for Christine – Final Update	http://CareforChristine.com
Memorial Sloan Kettering Cancer Center	http://mskcc.org
Be the Match (Bone Marrow Registry)	http://bethematch.org
Leukemia & Lymphoma Society	http://LLS.org
Team in Training (LLS Program)	http://teamintraining.org
Light the Night (LLS Program)	http://lightthenight.org
Steve Tornello (friend and creative genius)	http://stevetornello.com

ABOUT THE AUTHOR

Thomas Wonica grew up in Staten Island, NY. He graduated from Monsignor Farrell HS during which time he met his wife Christine. He attended Georgetown University in Washington, D.C. where he majored in computer science and was a 4 year member of the football team. Tom enjoys working with technology, acting, writing and working on projects. His favorite time is spent with his family. He cherishes the moments they spend together enjoying their second chance on life.

ABOUT THE SURVIVOR

Christine Wonica was born in Brooklyn, NY and moved to Staten Island while she was in the second grade. Christine was a standout softball player for most of her young life, eventually attending LIU Brooklyn on a full scholarship as a pitcher. Christine has a bachelor's degree in psychology and a master's degree in sports medicine from LIU. After her cure date, Christine began integrating herself back into normal activities as an elementary school teacher and coach. Most importantly, Christine has had the opportunity to watch her daughter Kailey grow up into a beautiful young woman who is preparing to attend college in the fall.